d.

88

MARGARET HILLS, SRN, trained at St Stephen's Hospital in London. She developed arthritis as a young woman, but despite predictions that she would never lead an active life she went on to finish her nurse's training, marry, have eight children and pursue a long career as an Industrial Nurse. She developed her own method of natural treatment for arthritis, and in 1982 she opened a clinic in Coventry. She has written two other books on the basis of her experience and success, *Curing Arthritis – The Drug-Free Way* and *Curing Arthritis Cookbook*, both published by Sheldon Press.

Overcoming Common Problems Series

The ABC of Eating
Coping with anorexia, bulimia and
compulsive eating
JOY MELVILLE

Acne
How it's caused and how to cure it
PAUL VAN RIEL

An A–Z of Alternative Medicine
BRENT Q. HAFEN AND KATHRYN J.
FRANDSEN

Arthritis
Is your suffering really necessary?
DR WILLIAM FOX

Birth Over Thirty
SHEILA KITZINGER

Body Language
How to read others' thoughts by their gestures
ALLAN PEASE

Calm Down
How to cope with frustration and anger
DR PAUL HAUCK

Comfort for Depression
JANET HORWOOD

Common Childhood Illnesses
DR PATRICIA GILBERT

Complete Public Speaker
GILES BRANDRETH

Coping Successfully with Your Child's Asthma
DR PAUL CARSON

Coping Successfuly with Your Hyperactive Child
DR PAUL CARSON

Coping with Depression and Elation
DR PATRICK McKEON

Curing Arthritis Cookbook
MARGARET HILLS

Curing Arthritis – The Drug-free Way
MARGARET HILLS

Depression
DR PAUL HAUCK

Divorce and Separation
ANGELA WILLANS

The Epilepsy Handbook
SHELAGH McGOVERN

Everything You Need to Know about Adoption
MAGGIE JONES

Everything You Need to Know about Contact Lenses
DR ROBERT YOUNGSON

Everything You Need to Know about Your Eyes
DR ROBERT YOUNGSON

Everything You Need to Know about the Pill
WENDY COOPER AND TOM SMITH

Everything You Need to Know about Shingles
DR ROBERT YOUNGSON

Family First Aid and Emergency Handbook
DR ANDREW STANWAY

Fears and Phobias
What they are and how to overcome them
DR TONY WHITEHEAD

Feverfew
A traditional herbal remedy for migraine and
arthritis
DR STEWART JOHNSON

Fight Your Phobia and Win
DAVID LEWIS

Fit Kit
DAVID LEWIS

Flying Without Fear
TESSA DUCKWORTH AND DAVID
MILLER

Overcoming Common Problems Series

Good Publicity Guide
REGINALD PEPLOW

Goodbye Backache
DR DAVID IMRIE WITH COLLEEN DIMSON

How to Bring Up your Child Successfully
DR PAUL HAUCK

How to Control your Drinking
DRS W. MILLER AND R. MUNOZ

How to Cope with Stress
DR PETER TYRER

How to Cope with your Child's Allergies
DR PAUL CARSON

How to Cope with your Nerves
DR TONY LAKE

How to Cope with Tinnitus and Hearing Loss
DR ROBERT YOUNGSON

How to Do What You Want to Do
DR PAUL HAUCK

How to Enjoy Your Old Age
DR B. F. SKINNER AND M. E. VAUGHAN

How to Improve Your Confidence
DR KENNETH HAMBLY

How to Interview and Be Interviewed
MICHELE BROWN AND GYLES BRANDRETH

How to Love a Difficult Man
NANCY GOOD

How to Love and be Loved
DR PAUL HAUCK

How to Say No to Alcohol
KEITH McNEILL

How to Sleep Better
DR PETER TYRER

How to Stand up for Yourself
DR PAUL HAUCK

How to Start a Conversation and Make Friends
DON GABOR

How to Stop Feeling Guilty
DR VERNON COLEMAN

How to Stop Smoking
GEORGE TARGET

How to Stop Taking Tranquillisers
DR PETER TYRER

If Your Child is Diabetic
JOANNE ELLIOTT

Jealousy
DR PAUL HAUCK

Learning to Live with Multiple Sclerosis
DR ROBERT POVEY, ROBIN DOWIE AND GILLIAN PRETT

Living with Grief
DR TONY LAKE

Living Through Personal Crisis
ANN KAISER STEARNS

Living with High Blood Pressure
DR TOM SMITH

Loneliness
DR TONY LAKE

Making Marriage Work
DR PAUL HAUCK

Making the Most of Yourself
GILL COX AND SHEILA DAINOW

Making Relationships Work
CHRISTINE SANDFORD AND WYN BEARDSLEY

Meeting People is Fun
How to overcome shyness
DR PHYLLIS SHAW

Overcoming Common Problems Series

No More Headaches
LILIAN ROWEN

One Parent Families
DIANA DAVENPORT

Overcoming Tension
DR KENNETH HAMBLY

The Parkinson's Disease Handbook
DR RICHARD GODWIN-AUSTEN

Second Wife, Second Best?
Managing your marriage as a second wife
GLYNNIS WALKER

Self-Help for your Arthritis
EDNA PEMBLE

The Sex Atlas
DR ERWIN HAEBERLE

Six Weeks to a Healthy Back
ALEXANDER MELLEBY

Solving your Personal Problems
PETER HONEY

A Step-Parent's Handbook
KATE RAPHAEL

Stress and your Stomach
DR VERNON COLEMAN

Trying to Have a Baby?
Overcoming infertility and child loss
MAGGIE JONES

What Everyone Should Know about Drugs
KENNETH LEECH

Why Be Afraid?
How to overcome your fears
DR PAUL HAUCK

You and Your Varicose Veins
DR PATRICIA GILBERT

Your Arthritic Hip and You
GEORGE TARGET

Overcoming Common Problems

CURING ILLNESS –
THE DRUG-FREE WAY

Margaret Hills, SRN

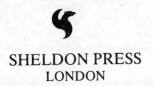

SHELDON PRESS
LONDON

First published in Great Britain in 1988 by
Sheldon Press, SPCK, Marylebone Road, London NW1 4DU

British Library Cataloguing in Publication Data

Hills, Margaret
    Curing illness: the drug-free way.—
    (Overcoming common problems).
    1. Naturopathy
    I. Title   II. Series
    615.5'35   RZ440

    ISBN 0–85969–561–1
    ISBN 0–85969–562–X Pbk

Photoset by Deltatype Ltd, Ellesmere Port
Printed in Great Britain by
Richard Clay Ltd, Bungay, Suffolk

For my children,
Michael, Christine, Graham, Sally, Clive, Peter,
Bill and Mary, and their children.

Acknowledgements

My sincere thanks go to my daughter Christine, and my daughter-in-law Jane, for the help they have given me in typing this book. My thanks also go to Mr Graham Shaw who very kindly contributed his report on my daughter Mary's illness and successful treatment.

Contents

Introduction   1

1 Coughs and Colds   3

2 Stomach Problems   15

Ulcers   15
Cancer   16
Diabetes   17
Colic   19
Diarrhoea   21
Constipation   23
Biliousness   26
Obesity   27

3 Circulatory and Other Problems   30

Varicose Veins   30
Piles   31
Anaemia   32
Thrush   34
Cystitis   35

4 Skin Problems   37

Nettle Rash   37
Eczema   38
Dermatitis   38
Acne   39
Boils   40
Dandruff   42
Baldness   42
Scabies   43

5   Diseases of the Muscles and Nerves   45

Strains 45
Rheumatism   46
Backache 47
Cramp   49
Heart Disease   52
Sleeplessness   56
Hiccough   57
Dizziness   57
Nervous Breakdown   58

6   Fevers   61

Measles   62
Scarlet Fever   63
Whooping Cough   64
Mumps   66
Chicken Pox   66
German Measles   66

7   Arthritis   68

8   Natural First Aid   75

9   The Value of Supplements   81

Conclusion   93

Appendix 1   Recommended Daily
    Requirements of Vitamins and
    Minerals   94

Appendix 2   Vitamins and Food   95

Index   97

Introduction

Since opening my arthritis clinic and the publication of my first book, *Curing Arthritis—The Drug-Free Way*, letters arrive day after day asking if I treat other ailments apart from arthritis the natural way. Also very often perhaps a husband will bring his wife along to the clinic for an appointment, and because she is getting such good results with her arthritis, he will ask me if I can do anything for his anaemia, angina or whatever. I say yes, certainly, and before long I have a whole family on my files, being treated naturally for ordinary, everyday ailments. I also treat my arthritis patients for other complaints they may suffer from, such as varicose veins, coughs, colds and flu. The number of these enquiries keep increasing, and over the years I have realized that people need to be taught how to deal with the ordinary illnesses that occur in the family. As most of these illnesses are due to wrong feeding, and of course you are what you eat, I decided to put together a collection of remedies to help the layman to help himself—the natural way.

In my opinion orthodox medical people are excellent at diagnosing and conquering infectious diseases, and of course our surgeons are invaluable, but not every problem can be solved by their methods. Cancer is a problem yet unsolved, and of course after many years of research no drug has been found to cure arthritis. I think a lot can be done to prevent, and in some cases cure, these chronic illnesses, and the letters I receive day by day from arthritic patients thanking me for bringing about their freedom from arthritic pain, migraine, thrush and so on prove to me that the natural way works, and works without any side effects. Unfortunately, drugs create very undesirable side effects—and these are sometimes worse than the disease itself. Some drugs are good if used discriminatingly, but if used indiscriminately they can be very dangerous—even the simple aspirin can cause nausea, vomiting and intestinal bleeding in some people.

As a State Registered Nurse Practitioner, I feel it is my duty to

1

convey to the public the facts about natural medicines and how effective they can be in the treatment of most illnesses. At the moment people tend to turn to them as a last resort, when conventional medicines have failed, or produce too many adverse side effects. In my view the opposite should be true, and the natural approach should be the first resort, and I can see no reason why holistic, complementary medicine should not become normal practice in the National Health system— alongside the proper use of drugs it could lead to a dramatic improvement in general health and save vast amounts of money.

As a nurse practitioner running a very busy clinic for arthritics, day after day patients relate to me the undesirable experiences they have had when given antibiotics and other drugs for various illnesses, particularly arthritis. These experiences have frightened them, and those that can afford it are now seeking natural relief from their ailments at my clinic; but for some it is too late—the damage is done and cannot be reversed. Those that come in time get wonderful results with holistic treatment, and before long they show signs of good health. Because they have been counselled on diet and nutrition, and shown the way to healthy living, their health continues to improve. These patients go on their way absolute converts to holistic medicine and so grateful that somebody recommended them to give it a try.

Natural medicines are prescribed in an atmosphere of increasing patient knowledge. The patient is told why he is given the medicine and how it actually works, and the medicine is prescribed on the basis of detailed personal knowledge. There is no known case of an adverse reaction report on any licensed natural medicine and many patients resort to natural medicine to avoid the addiction to prescribed synthetic drugs. More and more patients now want complementary medicine available from their doctor, and some doctors are—unofficially so far—offering their patients a variety of treatments. Until this desirable state of affairs becomes more widespread we can at least help ourselves with the ordinary everyday health problems that confront us, and in the following chapters I shall endeavour to give the reader some simple natural remedies that will promote good health, thereby making life easier for one and all.

1

Coughs and Colds

In my opinion, colds, bronchitis and bronchial troubles, coughs, asthma and pneumonia are mostly the result of a bad diet. Some of these conditions, such as colds and coughs, can be treated simply by these methods. Others are too serious not to be under medical care, but a lot can be done naturally to minimize the symptoms.

Colds

A cold is a catarrhal inflammation of the nose and upper respiratory passages, characterized by a feeling of chilliness, sneezing, watery eyes, watering nose and general discomfort. It usually lasts 10–14 days. Very often a condition known as herpes simplex or cold sores also occurs—watery blisters round the corners of the mouth and nose. These usually dry up and disappear in a week or two, and dabbing them with spirit is a good idea.

Most colds are due to a virus and are very infectious—if one member of the family gets one, everybody gets it. If a person is under par generally and resistance is low, frequent colds may ensue, bringing about a more debilitating effect still on the unfortunate sufferer, and in this case the cause should be investigated and removed if possible—it may be due to the adenoids or deformities of the nose or throat. Of course prevention is the best course and if you are susceptible and you feel a cold coming on you should make an immediate start by taking 600 milligrams of bioflavonoids and 600 milligrams of Vitamin C daily to prevent its occurrence.

A cold usually lasts between 7 and 10 days, and it is a consoling thought that during the watery stage a lot of acids are eliminated from the body. Because of this the patient's general health will be a lot better afterwards than before. Try to have a few days in bed,

3

especially if the cold is severe, and do not go to work—nobody will thank you for spreading it round the office. If you have a temperature, it is imperative that you go to bed. Take plenty of fresh fruit juices, but no food, and drink plenty of water; this regime will clear the system out and a quick return to good health will be the outcome. Do not worry about this starvation period—your body will be very grateful for the rest from food and a wonderful feeling of well–being will follow. Keep your bedroom well ventilated, as there is nothing worse than a stuffy room—it does nothing for the patient's outlook and only helps germs to multiply.

During the catarrhal stage, when your eyes and nose run, I have found Olbas oil invaluable. One or two drops on your tissue and inhaled clears the passages straight away. If the sinuses are blocked and painful a little of the oil rubbed gently across the forehead and along both sides of the nose, following the route of congestion and pain, will bring a lot of relief. Putting a tissue soaked in Olbas oil on your pillow to breathe in during the night will also help.

When you return to good health a well-balanced diet, sufficient rest, and proper dress both indoors and out all help to keep the body resistance high. You should take particular care to avoid people who have colds. Proper ventilation of rooms with sufficient humidity in the air helps to keep the mucous membranes in a healthy condition. If humidifiers are not used, adequate moisture can be maintained by keeping a container of water on a stove or radiator.

Sometimes in a cold you also have soreness of the throat, in which case gargling with salt and water—1 teaspoon salt to $\frac{1}{2}$ glass of warm water, three times daily—can be very beneficial. I have also found that 1 dessertspoon of cider vinegar in $\frac{1}{2}$ glass of warm water is excellent. Gargle with this three times daily and last thing at night. Also a drink of cider vinegar and honey three times daily will help give energy and restore the normal acid/alkaline balance in the body. Dissolve one teaspoon honey in a glass of hot water, add to this 2 teaspoons cider vinegar and stir—more honey may be taken if desired.

4

Exercise

Daily exercise is very important once the acute stage of the cold has passed. The right amount of the right type of exercise results in all parts of the body working at their best. The heart works efficiently, pumping the blood round the body and dealing with increased output as the occasion demands. The lungs also function well, providing an increased amount of oxygen when required. The increased amount of energy used in exercise ensures that the food you eat is metabolized, so that the digestive tract is not overloaded with unnecessary food and thereby functions better, as does the liver. Stresses and strains are minimized because the reflexes become brisker and the muscles are able to respond more effectively. There is also a deep satisfaction with life and, at the end of the day, the physical tiredness combined with emotional peace of mind brings about a deep, sound sleep.

If children do not get adequate exercise, slouching, faulty posture and flabbiness of the muscles may occur. Sometimes this may lead to curvature of the spine, and very often it is accompanied by mental lethargy. Sometimes these children do not use their lungs to their full breathing capacity, thereby starving the blood and cells of the body of adequate oxygen. This in turn can lead to lung disease, and the appetite becomes very poor and the skin is dull and pale. As these children grow into adults, and particularly when they reach middle age, lack of exercise leads to obesity with all its side-effects; which include varicose veins, coronary heart disease, breathlessness, hardening of the arteries and sometimes severe mental disturbances. I hope I have impressed upon the reader the importance of exercise for all ages.

Acute Bronchitis or Bronchial Catarrh

Bronchitis is an inflammation of the tubes in the lungs. It is one of the commonest diseases of our climate, and most prevalent in the winter months. It is usually the very young and the very old who suffer from it. An acute attack lasts only a few days or at most a week, whereas the chronic form persists for months and may recur again and again.

In the majority of cases the cause is exposure to cold and wet, especially in those who live or work in warm, badly-ventilated rooms. People who suffer from some other chronic disease are also at risk, and so are those run down by overwork or a poor diet.

Symptoms

Bronchitis varies greatly in severity from a mere cold and cough to a condition in which the patient has to fight for breath. In mild cases only the large bronchial tubes are affected, but in more severe cases the inflammation may attack the capillary tubes and sometimes the lung tissue may be affected, and this is broncho-pneumonia. Usually the first symptom is an irritating watery flow from the nose and eyes with frequent attacks of sneezing, sore throat and husky voice. The patient feels hot and feverish and out of sorts—the temperature may be raised slightly and the pulse is usually quicker than normal. Sometimes the limbs ache and the patient seems to have a chill all over. The cough usually comes on in fits. At first there is very little expectoration and what there is is thin and frothy in appearance, but after a time it becomes thicker and sometimes takes on a yellowish colour. If the inflammation extends to the small tubes the patient may get violent shivering fits, severe headache and vomiting, shortness of breath and rapid breathing may also occur, accompanied by loud wheezing. Sometimes the cough may be continuous and the temperature may rise to 103°F (39·5°C) or higher.

Treatment

During mild attacks the patient should be kept in bed in a warm, well-ventilated room. A hot bath may be taken immediately before going to bed, or the feet bathed in hot water, and the bed should first be warmed either with an electric blanket or hot water bottles. The patient should have a hot drink, preferably 2 teaspoons of honey dissolved in hot water with 2 teaspoons of cider vinegar. If the chest is sore it may be rubbed with camphorated oil or Vick or Olbas oil. (This is a blend including clove, eucalyptus, juniper and peppermint oils, and is available from all health food shops.) The addition of a little eucalyptus oil or Friars' Balsam to a bowl of very hot water and inhaled is excellent for loosening the phlegm. If the condition gets no better after a few days the doctor should be called in to make a proper diagnosis of the condition. The diet should be limited to fluids—water, fresh orange juice, honey and cider vinegar drinks—as long as the fever persists. Vitamin C should be given—2 grams per day and a cough mixture, made up as follows:

Add $\frac{1}{2}$ a spanish onion cut finely to $\frac{1}{2}$ a jar of clear honey, leave to soak over night and then strain. One desertspoonful to be taken three times daily.

This is by far the best cough mixture I know, as the onion is a natural antibiotic and the honey a natural energy giver.

A hot epsom salts bath may be taken daily—add three teacups of epsom salts to a bath of water as hot as you can bear—the patient soaks in this for approximately 10 minutes and then gets straight into his warm bed. The patient will probably sweat during the night, but will have a good restful night's sleep. A shower in the morning will clean away the perspiration and give a feeling of new awakening. This bath draws the congestion away from the lungs and tremendous relief is obtained from coughing and in breathing. Epsom salts may be bought from a chemist or garden centre.

As the fever subsides and convalescence begins, a return to a normal diet may be introduced by giving a little chicken broth, vegetable broth or a beaten egg in warmed, skimmed milk, then a little poached or grilled fish, chicken or a poached egg. The tendency to recur is very characteristic of bronchitis and should be carefully guarded against. Every possible precaution must be taken against catching cold—by wearing warm clothes (two layers of thin clothing is better than one thick layer), by breathing through the nose and, except for the aged, by toning up the skin daily by a cold sponge bath, beginning with tepid water to avoid shock to the system. A good quality multivitamin should be taken daily and also 500 mg vitamin C and 2 teaspoons of cod liver oil. Sometimes in children bronchitis is associated with whooping cough, with fevers or with constitutional diseases, and in such cases the catarrh may be long-term, with the child suffering from a persistent cough, and having some difficulty in breathing for weeks or months. Or the catarrh may develop into asthma or the bronchial tubes may be permanently enlarged and undergo ulceration—all such cases are serious and treatment should be directed by the doctor. However, the adoption of the treatment and prevention for acute bronchitis mentioned above will greatly help the situation and a recurrence of the problem may be guarded against by an abundance of nourishing food, taking the vitamins and minerals mentioned above, cold sponging, avoiding of over heated rooms and having plenty of fresh air and exercise. A daily intake of garlic capsules could be invaluable as this is an excellent blood cleanser, and it is absolutely imperative not to smoke and to avoid smoky atmospheres.

Chronic Bronchitis

A great many people suffer from a mild form of chronic bronchitis without knowing it. They begin the winter with a cough and keep it until the return of spring and this may happen regularly year after year. They speak of not being able to get rid of this dreadful cough, but really they are victims of chronic bronchitis, and it might be some comfort to them to know it. The symptoms are those of a mild case of bronchitis as described above. In certain cases this is called dry bronchitis, because although there is violent coughing the expectoration is scanty and is only expelled with difficulty as small pearly masses. In other cases the expectoration is abundant, and often there is shortness of breath. The bronchial tubes may in time come to be dilated, and this is called bronchiectasis. Sometimes, through repeated, violent coughing, the air sacs of the lungs may become distended and rupture—this is called emphysema.

Treatment

All that has been said in the preceeding article about the avoidance of cold applies with double force to persons who have long suffered with chronic bronchitis. Gentle walking in the fresh air is most important, and so are deep breathing exercises to help expand the lungs. The avoidance of dairy foods—butter, cheese, milk and cream—and of red meats, primarily pork and beef, is a must. Plenty of vegetables should be eaten raw if possible and lots of fruit, excluding particularly acid fruits such as oranges, lemons, tangerines, rhubarb and plums. A hot epsom salts bath may be taken 2–3 times per week, always immediately before retiring. (See p. 7) For those who are too weak to adopt these baths rubbing the back and chest with camphorated oil, Vick or Olbas oil will help enormously. Again the taking of good food, a good multivitamin, zinc, vitamin C and garlic should prove invaluable.

It is good to remember that coughs, colds and bronchitis are an attempt by the body to eliminate toxins that have accumulated, and that when the elimination process is complete and a return to normal health achieved naturally (without the use of drugs) the feeling of well-being experienced will be so much better than if you have resorted to the use of drugs, with all their side effects.

Bronchial Asthma

Sometimes asthma may accompany bronchitis and it can happen at a very early age. Sudden attacks of shortness of breath is at first noticed, and this is more frequent in boys. Children of parents who have suffered from asthma are apt to inherit a susceptibility to it. Bronchial asthma is due to a spasm of the muscle fibres in the walls of the smaller tubes in the lungs. A child suffering from a cold in the chest may be suddenly seized with breathlessness and these breathless attacks may continue intermittently. It is a very distressing condition for the child, and just as distressing for the parents to watch their child in that condition. During an attack suddenly plunging the child into a warm bath may do much to relieve the breathlessness. The doctor should be called and warm drinks given.

Treatment

The child should be allowed to live a free, active life, get as much fresh air as possible, always sleep in a well-ventilated room, and care must be taken that his physical and mental capacities are not overtaxed. A good dietary regime should be followed, with plenty of fresh fruit and vegetables and wholemeal bread, and cakes. Honey is invaluable and should be given daily, as it fills in any gaps that may occur in the daily food intake and it is an excellent source of potassium. Honey also calms the nerves, gives a good nights sleep and is very soothing to the stomach. It is a wonderful source of energy, a gentle laxative and very easily and quickly absorbed by the body. It contains a lot of vitamins, especially the all-important vitamin C, which can so easily be destroyed in cooking. A good multivitamin should be given each day and a proper daily routine adhered to.

There are various types of asthma, which include cardiac asthma from heart disease, renal asthma from kidney disease and others, and what is known as allergic asthma. This may be caused by the inhalation of pollens or emanations from the fur of cats or dogs or from eating white of egg or some other food. Sometimes to some people the mere suggestion that they are exposed to the cause of their asthma is enough to bring on an attack. In all cases the adoption of a well ordered life, good, nourishing food, plenty of fresh air and as much exercise as can easily be taken is the only way to avoid attacks and build resistance to the complaint.

I should like to recount here my own experience with my youngest child, Mary. She was bonny, dark haired with large brown eyes. Everybody remarked on the lovely-looking child, always happy and playful and thoroughly spoiled by her older brothers and sisters—she was the youngest of eight.

About two months after she started nursery school she developed a persistent cough which continued in spite of a visit to the doctor and a course of antibiotics. Then she developed a temperature which was brought down for 24 hours by a different antibiotic only to escalate even higher than before. By now Mary's illness had been diagnosed as bronchial asthma and recurrent attacks of pneumonia—and her condition was worsening by the day. Another antibiotic was tried but to no avail, and our doctor was really baffled. Mary was finding it increasingly difficult to breathe, and now the infection had spread and her right lung collapsed completely. She lost a tremendous amount of weight in that month, and went from the healthy, fun-loving child we knew to an irritable, frail little girl who could not sleep or eat and who was too weak to sit or walk. A further rise in temperature brought the doctor once more and this time he suggested that Mary be admitted to hospital for tests. This was to prove quite an ordeal for me, because Mary needed me with her in hospital and of course the other children needed me at home.

However, somehow we managed and each morning, having prepared the others for school, I would make my way to the hospital to be with Mary. The children's specialist was wonderful, and he did every test imaginable, but all proved negative. Mary got worse and worse, until when she had spent a month in hospital he told me that he could do no more and now we could only pray for recovery—which I had been doing since she first became ill. I asked the specialist if I might take her home, and he said I could if I wanted to. Being a State Registered Nurse I knew I had nothing to lose.

She had been at home two days when there was a sudden dramatic rise in temperature which necessitated calling in the specialist—only to have him confirm his former statement that there was nothing he could do. Knowing that the medical profession could do nothing for her I decided to contact an alternative medical practitioner called Mr Shaw. He is a registered naturopath and osteopath, although in those days such people were regarded as 'quacks'. He arrived that evening and having spent two hours taking Mary's case history, going into every detail of her illness and family history he turned to me and said, 'I'll save Mary for you, Mrs Hills, but you must do exactly as I say'. This of course I promised. He said firstly we should put Mary on a diet of grapes only for ten days to get rid of the antibiotics, to give him a firm foundation to build on. Now Mr Shaw, who very kindly contributed his report at my request takes up the story:

I well remember being called to see a young child, Miss Mary Hills, to be greeted by her distraught, loving mother who was also a well-qualified nurse, and her father who was decidedly opposed to any 'quack' treatment by an 'unqualified' individual.

In this atmosphere I was asked if I could do anything for their daughter, who was suffering from recurrent attacks of pneumonia. After examination and assessment of the history and present symptoms, I considered that nature could produce a recovery, but I insisted that the mother must adhere strictly and precisely to the instructions given. Success or failure would depend entirely on this.

I issued instructions for cold water body packs to be given, and I told Mrs Hills to check carefully that a warm reaction was produced within ten minutes of application. I also instructed that before this the patient should take a hot infusion of herbal tea, which included such items as pleurisy root, liquorice, yarrow and mousear, with marigold and lily of the valley for heart support, designed to stimulate the blood circulation to ensure the above mentioned warm reaction of the pack. A medicine of similar ingredients was prescribed to be taken several times daily.

The net result of this treatment was that the symptoms eased and the patient felt much better. The intervals between recurrences of the illness became longer and longer, until at last the condition was eliminated.

As a sequel to this I might add that Mary spent some years as games captain of her form at school, she has excelled at karate and is now a happily married, joyful, healthy girl of 22.

The step-by-step counselling given to me to enable me to understand the treatment procedure in Mary's illness was invaluable and has had an effect on me and my treatment of all members of my family ever since. That success in the face of all medical opinions, plus the fact that in my own arthritis natural methods of healing triumphed where drugs failed, have helped to convert me to exploring natural treatment first in every case of illness. At the moment people tend to turn to natural medicines as a last resort, when conventional medicines are either in-effective or produce too many adverse reactions. In my view the opposite should be true. If people explored natural medicine first, there would be a considerable reduction in the queues in doctors' surgeries and great savings could be made. In Britain alone the cost of synthetic drugs taken today runs at £2 billion per year and manufacturers of synthetic drugs spend about £30,000 per year per doctor in marketing their medicines, and there is now one drug company representative for every eight doctors.

It is estimated that 75% of all consultations end in the prescription of a synthetic drug, but at least 40% of patients never take their drugs. Adverse drug reactions are grossly under-reported, but even so about 4,000 deaths in the UK each year are officially attributed to prescribed drugs, which are known as 'therapeutic misadventures'. The cost to the health service in Britain of drug-induced illness is impossible to estimate but it must be quite considerable, for many hospital beds are occupied by patients suffering from the side-effects of various drugs. I hope I have impressed upon the reader the great necessity for investigating a natural line of approach every time, before trying the doctor's surgery.

Pneumonia

There are two types of pneumonia—lobar, where the whole of one or both of the lobes of the lung are involved, and broncho-pneumonia, where the disease is confined to smaller sub-divisions of the lung tissue. When the word pneumonia is used it is usually broncho-pneumonia that is meant. It is sometimes known as catarrhal pneumonia.

Broncho-pneumonia usually begins as bronchitis and spreads to the tissues of the lungs. The symptoms are similar to those of acute bronchitis but much more pronounced—breathing is rapid and difficult, the pulse is weak and quick, the cough is persistent and violent and the fluid coughed up is thick and sometimes streaked with blood. Diarrhoea and vomiting often occurs and often the patient is very thirsty. The temperature may go up to 104°F (40°C). Recovery is very gradual and sometimes may be incomplete, leaving the patient with some form of lung disease.

Treatment

A doctor should be called and a proper diagnosis made, but a tremendous amount can be done to relieve the symptoms. For instance, to bring down the temperature sponging with tepid or cold water is usually sufficient. If the pulse is feeble and breathing becomes strained, a little brandy in water can help a lot. The inhalation of steam referred to in acute bronchitis is invaluable and rubbing the chest with Vick, camphorated oil or Olbas oil will bring a lot of relief. As convalescence begins a good, light but nourishing diet should be adopted, along the lines of the diet suggested for asthma in this chapter.

2

Stomach Problems

In this chapter I will deal with disorders which affect the stomach. Many of these are caused by a faulty diet, and can be helped by adopting a wholefood diet and healthy lifestyle, and taking vitamin supplements.

Stomach ulcers

These are mainly due to the formation of too much acid in the stomach. In almost all cases there is a burning sensation or stabbing or cramping pain. Sometimes there is a feeling of nausea followed by vomiting; bleeding may also occur. In addition to the pain there is often a feeling of weight in the pit of the stomach, with flatulence (wind) and the bringing up of extremely acid fluid. The most serious is gastric ulcer—the patient feels a sudden and agonizing pain and may even collapse. Of course in such severe cases a doctor must be called and a proper diagnosis made, but a lot can be done by the patient to relieve his own symptoms. Worry is a prime factor in the cause of stomach ulcers, so all stress should be avoided. People with arthritis often suffer from stomach ulcers because the body contains too much acid, so day by day in the running of my clinic I meet a lot of such sufferers, and as soon as I put them on my acid-free diet they seem to improve tremendously. This diet is described in detail in the chapter on arthritis, pages 68–73.

Treatment

The patient should go to bed, and rest the body in general and the stomach in particular. To give the ulcer a chance to heal nothing but boiled water and skimmed milk should be given. Small quantities of chicken broth or veal broth may be added gradually, but everything should be given in small quantities— one tablespoon every hour, increasing to a teacupful every two or three hours. Later, beaten eggs may be given and then a very gradual adoption of the acid-free diet referred to earlier for arthritics. Duodenal ulcers produce symptoms similar to gastric ulcers and require the same treatment.

Colitis

This is inflammation of the colon, at the end of the digestive system, and it can be caused by too much uric acid in the body and by eating indigestible, irritating foods or unripe fruit. There may be a rise in temperature, loss of appetite, headache, furred tongue and pain all over the abdomen, and in some cases jaundice may occur. If the lower bowel is affected there is severe diarrhoea. As in all cases of acute inflammation of the bowel the patient should rest in bed and food should be limited to skimmed milk, chicken and veal broth and all drinks taken tepid. Later a wholefood, fibre-rich diet may be adopted gradually.

Diverticulitis

Diverticulitis is little pockets of ulcers in the colon which produce a similar set of symptoms. Again it is due to too much acid in the body. Taking vitamin A, which protects against ulcers and viral invasions of the digestive tract which cause diarrhoea and similar problems, is a very good idea. The recommended daily allowance for a healthy person is 5,000 international units daily, but 10,000–100,000 units may be taken. People deficient in this vitamin produce the following symptoms—night blindness, dry skin, loss of appetite, diarrhoea, ulcers, loss of hearing and very slow healing of cuts. Some people are also prone to a lot of infections.

Cancer of stomach or bowel

Early detection of cancer is absolutely necessary, so everybody who finds a lump, painful or not, should have it examined at once by the doctor, who will carry out tests to see whether or not it is malignant, or dangerous. Early diagnosis and the improvement of modern surgical techniques now lead to the possibility of operations which can considerably prolong life in a patient suffering from abdominal cancer. The patient suffering from cancer can do a great deal to help himself by the following methods:–

- A good wholesome diet should be adopted, and the patient should eat plenty of raw vegetables and fruits every day.
- Dairy foods should be omitted from the diet and the acid-free diet for arthritics adhered to. (See pages 68–73)
- Avoid all red meat.
- Large quantities of supplementary vitamins and minerals should be taken daily. These should include:

Calcium	1500 mg
Magnesium	500 mg
Potassium	100 mg
Zinc	100 mg
Iron	100 mg
Vitamin A	5000 International Units
B Complex	(which contains all the B vitamins) 50 mg
Vitamin C	10,000 mg
Vitamin D	400 International Units
Vitamin E	400 International Units

- Drink plenty of water.
- Take plenty of exercise in the fresh air.
- Don't smoke, and avoid smoky atmospheres.
- Last, but not least, adopt a positive attitude to your disease. Think positively—whatever is worrying you may never happen. Take one day at a time and always remember that a little prayer goes a long way towards calming the mind.

Diabetes

There are two kinds of diabetes—diabetes insipidus and diabetes mellitus, meaning honeyed or sweet diabetes. This is the type I am dealing with here and is the more common. It is characterized by the presence of sugar in the urine, although this in itself is not always an indication of diabetes, as it may be a temporary condition which is explained by an excessive consumption of sugary foods and which ceases as soon as the diet is modified. The cause of diabetes is due essentially to a deficiency of insulin in the body—insulin is the internal secretion of the pancreas which enables the body to use sugar for energy. When there is a deficiency of this substance in the body, the sugar in the blood is not properly disposed of but remains there until it is filtered out by the kidneys and carried off in the urine. When insulin is administered in such cases it causes a rapid reduction of the sugar in the urine and the blood.

Hereditary influence appears to play a big part in the cause of diabetes, and it occurs more often in men than women. When it occurs in the young, the symptoms appear rapidly and insulin production soon stops altogether. Insulin is usually given to regulate the condition. When diabetes occurs in middle age the symptoms come on gradually, presumably because the metabolism has slowed down, and they can often be treated by diet alone.

Symptoms

The urine is increased in quantity, it is clear and pale, and in many cases has a greenish tinge. One indication of the disease is the peculiar odour of the urine—like that of apples or new mown grass. If the urine is excessive in quantity the patient suffers from extreme thirst, the patient loses weight and strength and is easily fatigued. There is frequently great mental depression and irritability. In severe cases the skin becomes dry and harsh, the secretion of sweat almost ceases, there is great liability to eruptions and boils and gangrene may be set up by quite slight injuries, as for instance to one of the toes. The hair becomes thin and the nails brittle, the breath may have a sweet, heavy odour and the patient may be conscious of a sweet taste in the mouth. The motions are very hard and dry.

Treatment

Severe cases are always, nowadays, treated medically with insulin, which does not actually cure the disease but enables the patient to take in a certain amount of foods containing sugar or starch, although the quantities must be regulated. It controls the symptoms and enables the patient to work and otherwise function normally. Most patients suffering from diabetes are overweight, and less severe cases can be treated quite successfully with diet only. Sugar should be avoided, and the intake of starch limited because this is converted into sugar by the saliva and other gastric juices. The daily allowances of milk should be reduced, but all green vegetables are important in the diet and most animal foods can be eaten. It is very important to have a daily intake of chromium and zinc, as subnormal levels of these two minerals have been noted in patients suffering from this complaint. A supplement of 25 mg zinc and 15 mg chromium should be taken, with brewers' yeast and vitamins E, B6 and C. Patients suffering from diabetes should be careful to avoid chills, and should take gentle exercise every day.

Colic

Colic is a painful spasm in the gut, and the term is used to include all painful affections of the intestines not due to inflammation. Affections of other abdominal organs give rise to similar pain and may be mentioned here. The onset of inflammation of the bowels from twists, rupture, knots of the intestine etc., is accompanied by acute pain like colic, and so is the passage of kidney and gall stones. These can all be serious, so intense or prolonged colic should be a warning to obtain skilled medical advice.

In Children

Colic in children is most commonly due to flatulence from indigestible food, overfeeding, an inadequate diet either because of underfeeding or giving milk which is very poor in quality, whether human or cow's. Severe purgatives can also cause it. Constipation or diarrhoea usually accompanies the colic. The commonest cause is cow's milk insufficiently diluted, which causes big indigestible curds to form in the stomach.

Soon after taking food the child is restless, kicks, seems in

19

pain, draws up its legs, perhaps cries with usually a sharp piercing scream. It becomes pale, returns its food or belches wind. If the child is constipated there is much straining and hard, lumpy stools are passed, which may be a little blood-stained.

Treatment consists of applying gentle massage over the abdomen or heat in the form of hot flannels. Keep the child warm. If convulsions have occurred, as sometimes happens, a few drops of brandy in a little warm water should be given. If colic is associated with constipation half to one teaspoon of castor oil should be given and an enema administered. I always used Woodwards gripe water for my children—it worked wonders.

Colic in Adults

The causes of colic in adults are many. Intestinal irritants, coarse, indigestible foods, overeating, intense constipation, exposure to cold, lead poisoning, eating decomposing food, diseases of other abdominal organs, hysteria and certain nervous diseases, rupture of the intestine and appendicitis are some of them. Pains can either develop gradually with a feeling of sickness and flatulence, or it can be sudden and severe, doubling up the patient by its intensity, situated chiefly at the naval and shooting around the abdomen. The muscles of the abdomen become hard and knotted, and there is always restlessness and twisting of the body. Some sweating may occur.

It is very important to distinguish between simple colic and inflammation of the bowel. In inflammation there is fever, the pulse and breathing are fast and there is a rise in temperature. There is always thirst. Very slight pressure causes pain, and the patient is very quiet, very pale and anxious, nearly always vomiting, and keeps his legs drawn up to his stomach.

Complete fasting on boiled water only is necessary for 24 hours. If the condition is no better medical help should be called. If colic is habitual you should treat it as for constipation and attend to the diet. Avoid pastry, sweets, nuts and cheese and other indigestible foods.

Colic From Passage of Gall- and Kidney-Stones

Gall-stone colic is very severe and sets in suddenly with pain over the right side of the lower part of the chest and upper part of the abdomen and shooting to the right shoulder. There is a rise of temperature, and usually vomiting and profuse sweating with shivering or chill. It may be followed by jaundice.

Immediately give a hot bath or apply hot fomentations over the liver. Sipping hot water to which two teaspoons of bicarbonate of soda has been added can be very beneficial. If the colic persists, a doctor should be consulted.

Kidney colic is also sudden, but the pain may be in right or left loin, and it usually shoots down into the groin or thigh. The other symptoms are similar to gall-stone colic. Blood may appear in the urine before or soon after an attack, and the patient passes water frequently.

Diarrhoea

Diarrhoea often affects bottle-fed babies, particularly at the time of teething. It is caused by improper feeding and food, particularly by eating too much coarse and irritating food, especially unripe fruit, tainted milk, bad meat, fish of various kinds, and starchy foods given too early.

The attacks vary greatly from rather slight increase in the number of stools to sudden intense diarrhoea with great pain, abdominal swelling, vomiting and collapse, when the child shrinks noticeably in a few days. Sudden crying and drawing up of the legs is an invariable accompaniment of pain in the abdomen.

Treatment

Prevention is better than cure. Feed the child properly according to its age, and have all utensils scrupulously clean. To treat existing diarrhoea the following routine should be followed. If the stools contain undigested milk, or are very foul, sour or green in colour give ½–1 teaspoon of castor oil, to clear away any irritating material. It is best in severe cases to discontinue milk

21

entirely and just give tepid, boiled water in small quantities frequently, every half an hour if necessary. This rests the digestive system and allows a clearing out to take place. After 24 hours a gradual return to the normal meals should be acceptable. Sometimes a few drops of brandy added to water helps settle the stomach. Repeated washing out of the bowel through use of a plain water enema using half a pint of water, helps to clear the system. The child must be kept warm.

Chronic Diarrhoea

In chronic diarrhoea the cause is chiefly dietetic, especially over-eating and drinking or eating the wrong foods such as de-composing food, tinned meats, certain fish and poisons of various kinds. It can also be caused by

- Chronic Bright's disease or liver disease
- Sudden chill
- Constipation
- Nervousness or fear
- Infection by foul water
- Dysentery, typhoid fever and other serious diseases

Therefore if the diarrhoea is persistent a doctor should investigate the cause.

Treatment

Treatment consists of avoiding any irritating foods, or those which leave a lot of solids after digestion, such as green vegetables, nuts, unripe fruits, indigestible meats. Take boiled milk, arrowroot, sago, tapioca or ground rice. A couple of days after the diarrhoea has stopped you can gradually return to your ordinary diet, resuming puddings and jellies, white fish and mince and then chicken or lamb chop with a little boiled potato. Occasional enemas of soap and water can be very beneficial (see p. 25). In all forms of diarrhoea warmth to the body is absolutely essential and relieves the pain. A hot water bottle on the abdomen or a hot fomentation are especially useful. Rice carefully boiled in water then taken with a little salt as the only food for 48 hours—the boiled rice water should be drunk cold. This often cuts short an attack, especially when the diarrhoea is due to fruit or climatic influence, such as when you are on holiday abroad. Drink plenty of this rice water when you are thirsty. This is a common remedy in Italy.

Constipation

These are the commonest causes of constipation

- Foods that are too easily digested, especially milk, which leave little residue to excite the bowels to act. In other words lack of fibre in the diet.
- Insufficiency of fluids, making the residue too hard and dry.
- Sedentary habits and lack of exercise.
- A deficient amount of bile and other digestive juices.
- Too frequent drug taking, constant use of purgatives in endeavouring to treat the symptom while neglecting the cause.

The most common cause of constipation is to be found in the diet. In these days bread and other kinds of food are carefully divested of those coarser elements which cannot be assimilated (known as fibre) and the result is that the bowels, deprived of the stimulation which such substances would supply, become sluggish and inactive. In some cases the diet contains too little liquid, and the amount of fluid is insufficient to keep the contents of the intestinal canal soft. This deficiency may also arise from excessive exercise in persons who perspire freely. On the other hand, constipation may be due to lack of exercise. Yet another cause is inattention to the calls of nature. There are many cases of constipation, however, in which no neglect can be alleged against the sufferers. They may suffer from anaemia or some other affection which deprives the bowels of their tone; or there may be an insufficient secretion of bile. There are also many persons in whom the bowels are naturally inactive, so that it is only by constant attention to diet and exercise that the bowels may be made to move.

Constipation is nearly always associated with a coated tongue, a bad taste in the mouth, disordered digestion, flatulence, palpitation. Dark patches form under the eyes, spots appear before them, the face may be flushed, and there may be headache and giddiness. The sufferer becomes irritable, and is restless and drowsy or heavy, he may have deep but unrefreshing sleep or suffer from the opposite condition of sleeplessness and there is often great depression of spirit. The long-term effects of constipation are serious and numerous, and are partly due to pressure upon the vessels and nerves. These include anaemia, piles, varicose veins, varicocele, prolapse or descent of the lining of the rectum, sciatica, rupture through straining, colic fever, ulcers in the bowels which may cause peritonitis and appendicitis or diverticulitis.

Treatment

The treatment consists of correcting the diet. It is important to alter the balance between animal and vegetable foods. You should eat less butcher's meat, and eat instead poultry, fish, eggs and game, and eat more vegetables, such as lettuce, spinach, endive, seakale, asparagus, cauliflower, tomatoes, celery, peas, beans, watercress and onions. Salads dressed with oil and vinegar are to be recommended. Ripe fruits of all kinds should be taken regularly—prunes, figs, bananas, grapes, stewed pears and apples are especially good. Always eat wholemeal bread and cakes instead of those made with white flour. Avoid anything which, from experience, causes indigestion, and increase your fluid intake to about three pints a day. For breakfast take porridge well cooked, brown bread, with a little butter and marmalade. Half a pint of cold water should be taken slowly before breakfast. Ripe fruit before breakfast may be taken instead of water. All drinks at meals should always be sipped.

Moderate exercise should always be taken, preferably in the open air, but if not convenient exercise indoors should be performed. Golf is good for the elderly and walking is beneficial for all. For the young any form of exercise is helpful, if it is not too violent, and remember that if free perspiration is induced the intake of fluids should be increased.

24

Attention should be given to the natural desire to unload the bowel whenever it should occur. At a regular hour daily, an action of the bowel should be encouraged, preferably soon after breakfast. Avoid tight clothing about the abdomen which prevents free movement of the intestine. The misuse of purgatives is especially bad in habitual constipation. Patients constantly take powerful pills which relieve the bowel for a time but do not cure the problem, and they come to need increasing doses to give relief. Alternatively they take salines daily which wash out all the intestinal fluids, but leave the solids behind.

If changes in the diet and regular habits fail to solve the problem you may need to resort to aperients. Senna pods are a time-honoured remedy for constipation. Seven or eight pods are placed in half a tumbler of cold water in the morning, and the infusion, which has no taste, is drunk at bedtime. It may be taken for a time and discontinued when no longer necessary. Liquorice powder is another good aperient—a teaspoon of the powder is stirred in a little water and taken at night or in the morning.

How to give an enema

In very severe cases it may be necessary to use an enema. Enemas may consist of a pint of tepid water with or without soap. You can add an ounce of castor oil, though this is not usually necessary.

An enema apparatus can be bought at any chemists. You also need an enema can or container. The can containing the water should be suspended about three feet above the level of the buttock and the nozzle slightly lubricated with vaseline. The patient can then either lie on the left side or on the knees and elbows. The nozzle is then inserted into the rectum and the tap gently opened. The enema is retained for 10–15 minutes and then the bowel is unloaded. This ensures rapid and effective relief and avoids the uncertainty of purgatives. The daily use of enema ensures unloading of the bowel and by its use for a month or six weeks, combined with a good fibre-filled diet and general treatment, will cure constipation. If anaemia is present 500 mg of vitamin C and 50 mg of iron should be taken daily.

Constipation in Children

This can be due to a number of causes, such as taking too little exercise, eating too much animal food, or of neglecting to go to the toilet. Some cases, however, are associated with hysteria or some other manifestation of a nervous temperament. In the case of breast-fed infants the mother should eat plenty of green vegetables and fruit, and drink plenty of water. The baby's abdomen may be gently massaged. Suppositories of soap or glycerine jelly may be introduced into the lower bowel. Liquid paraffin should be taken in sufficient doses to prevent stools becoming hard—approximately ½ teaspoon twice daily, either taken alone or in milk or malt or honey. Should these measures fail, a gentle laxative must be used for a few days—1 or 2 senna pods may be infused and taken at bedtime. In older children, reliance should be placed upon dietary and hygenic habits. A fibre-rich diet is most important, incorporating plenty of green vegetables, fresh fruit and wholemeal bread. If constipation continues, in children or adults, you should consult your doctor.

Biliousness

This is a term applied either to migraine or to feelings of headache and nausea, sometimes with vomiting. It occurs when the liver is overloaded with bile. It is often associated with defective eye-sight and is frequently due to constipation. The symptoms are a feeling of weight and heaviness and intense depression, and a violent headache. In addition, the complexion is muddy or sallow, the white of the eyes slightly yellow and they look heavy and dull. Vomiting is a very frequent symptom and consists of bile-coloured stomach contents or pure bile, usually with painful retching. There may be a sense of weight or tenderness in the right side over the liver. The attacks are nearly always periodical, occuring once a fortnight or once a month.

Treatment

Prevention, as in constipation, is the best treatment. Have the eyes examined. During an attack avoid too much study or close eye work, rest, and don't eat solid food. A hot fomentation (see p. 45) over the pit of the stomach often relieves the discomfort and allays the vomiting. Taking stewed rhubarb has been known to be very beneficial in attacks due to constipation.

Obesity

An excessive development of adipose or fatty tissue throughout the body is called obesity. Besides accumulating in the anterior abdominal wall, the buttocks, the back and other superficial situations the fat collects over the internal organs such as the heart. A tendency to obesity may be noted in some families and in a considerable proportion of all individuals who have passed middle life. In certain cases obesity is due to lack of activity of glands of internal secretion, notably the thyroid, the pituitary, the testicle and the ovary. Fat in the body is derived mainly from carbohydrate foods, but may be formed from fats or proteins. Obesity may result, therefore, from consumption of an excessive amount of food especially when an insufficient amount of open air exercise is taken. Over-indulgence in liquors is a common cause of obesity. In some persons, usually women, the existence of anaemia accounts for obesity, as the tissues are not properly oxygenated.

An obese person tends to be short of breath on slight exertion. This happens because the heart loses its power to contract and may become dilated and very feeble. Many obese people also develop emphysema (see p. 8) and this is another cause of shortness of breath. Active exercise thus becomes difficult and the enforced sedentary habits increase the obesity. The bowels are sluggish, the liver is enlarged and is also sluggish, so the digestion may be poor and there is a tendency to gall-stones. Some people develop glycosuria (sugar in the urine, see diabetes, p. 17), others suffer from nephritis (inflammation of the kidneys).

Treatment

The treatment of obesity consists of a controlled diet and more exercise. The changes required in the diet are to cut down the carbohydrates, that is sugar and starches, to a minimum, to cut out all fat and restrict the total amount of food. No one diet is suitable for everybody because of varying life styles and varying metabolic rate. Before embarking on a weight-reducing diet, check with your doctor in case there is any hormone imbalance. Age is an important factor when reducing—a growing person requires a liberal amount of protein, whereas the daily amount of tissue waste in an adult is not very great, and hard work makes no appreciable difference—an increased amount of meat has no physiological justification.

The Balanced Diet

Three food constitutents should always be represented in the diet, namely proteins, carbohydrates and fats. It may be said that most people could do with less protein than is commonly taken. A larger intake of carbohydrate than fat should be taken when there is demand for more energy. Any good diet, reducing or otherwise, should also include mineral salts such as iron, calcium, magnesium, sodium, potassium and zinc. These are necessary in tissue building, and in various ways in the chemical processes which go on in the body; iron is a necessary constituent of red blood corpuscles, for example, and calcium of bone, while sodium chloride (salt) is a constituent of blood and the source of hydrochloric acid in the gastric juices. The diet should also include vitamins—the most commonly known being as follows:–

Vitamin A which prevents eye problems in particular
Vitamin B complex which is very necessary for nerve health and function
Vitamin C which prevents scurvy
Vitamin D which prevents rickets
Vitamin E which is necessary for reproduction and the health of the heart and arteries

And of course no diet is complete without zinc and fibre. Zinc nourishes the immune system, helping to fight off various illnesses. It is amazing how many people today are lacking in zinc—white spots on the nails are a good indication of a lack of zinc. Fibre helps the action of the bowel, helping elimination which is a very important part of digestion. It is possible that many ill-defined diseases occurring in those who feed on artificial foods and follow crash diets are explained by vitamin deficiency. Any weight-reducing diet should be under the guidance of a specialist backed up by all possible information on the person's health.

3

Circulatory and Other Problems

Varicose veins, piles and varicose ulcers are circulatory problems, and as in the previous chapters a good diet plays a big part
in their prevention. Plenty of exercise is also important, as
sluggish circulation is their main cause. Thrush and vaginal
itching can be caused by taking antibiotics or a rundown digestive
system, and the treatment is explained under the individual
headings.

Varicose Veins

Varicose veins are veins in which the valves don't function
properly so blood collects, and they are most often seen as blue
lumps on the legs. People who do a great deal of standing are
mostly prone to this condition. Other causes are the use of tight
garters, habitual constipation and congestion of the liver.

Varicose veins may not cause any trouble, but usually an
aching pain is felt in the leg, often accompanied by a sense of
weight and fullness, and sometimes by numbness and weakness.
The feet are always cold and after walking or a hard days work
the ankles are liable to swell. The dangers to be feared from
varicose veins are firstly that as a result of exertion or a slight
accident the vein may burst, and secondly that a clot of blood
may become detached and be carried along in the blood stream
until it blocks a channel too small for it to pass through. It then
cuts off the blood supply to the part of the body where its
progress is checked.

Treatment

Should constipation be the cause it should be treated as I have
described earlier (pages 24–25). If the problem is caused by
wearing tight garters this must be stopped. If the person is
overweight a slimming down process should be adopted. If on

the other hand the patient is ill-nourished a good high-fibre diet should be adopted, coupled with a good multivitamin and 400 international units of vitamin E and 500 mg of lecithin. An elastic stocking should be worn, and you should put it on as you get out of bed. In many cases these measures are sufficient to stop the symptoms becoming worse, and early treatment will prevent varicose ulcers from developing.

Piles

Piles, or haemorrhoids, consist of dilated and varicose veins at the anus or in the lower inch or two of the rectum. An external pile is sometimes formed, and it may cause no trouble at all, except perhaps a little itching or a sense of tightness when the bowels are moved. Internal piles may consist of thickened folds, or of rounded masses with something like a stalk covered with mucous membrane, which is a reddish-blue colour. The first variety is apt to cause prolapse—or falling down of the lining of the bowel so that it protrudes through the anus; the second variety are likely to prolapse themselves and also cause bleeding, sometimes to a serious extent.

Internal piles sometimes become inflamed and the blood in the veins may clot, and these occurrences give rise to considerable pain and distress. Sometimes the pile can get strangulated by the sphincter muscle in the rectum, which makes it swell up and become very painful and tender. An external pile may also become inflamed, and form a bluish swelling which is painful and tender.

Piles may be caused by chronic constipation, too much sitting about or the pressure of a pregnant womb.

Treatment

When piles exist, internal or external, it is important to correct any constipation. No strong purgatives should be used however. The anal region must be kept very clean, and it should be washed after every bowel movement. A little witch-hazel ointment should be smeared around the anus if there is any irritation. Care

31

should be taken against getting wet and cold, and cold seats should be avoided. If an external pile becomes inflamed, bed rest for a day or two is desirable, and the bowels should be opened thoroughly by means of a large enema (see p. 25). The use of hot fomentations (see p. 45) may cause the inflammation to subside. Daily exercise is very important and so is a high-fibre diet containing plenty of raw fruits and vegetables. Vitamin E and lecithin supplements should also be taken—400 international units of vitamin E and 500 mg lecithin every day.

Anaemia

The word anaemia means bloodlessness or 'poverty of the blood'. This phrase does not quite cover all the ground, for anaemic symptoms may be the result of a diminution of the volume of the blood as a profuse haemorrhage, but in most instances anaemia means a reduction either in the number of red corpuscles or in their red colouring matter, which is called haemoglobin. In the one case there are too few red corpuscles; in the other the red corpuscles are not red enough. The phrase 'poverty of the blood' is not, therefore, very wide of the mark. Anaemia may be secondary to many other conditions, or it may be a primary disease—a disease by itself.

Primary anaemia occurs chiefly in girls, especially between the ages of fourteen and seventeen. It is closely associated with sexual development and with irregularities of menstruation. Lack of sunshine, working or living in poorly ventilated places, an insufficiency of nourishing food, and the absorption of poisons from the intestine in cases of constipation are also believed to promote anaemia. It is now much less frequent than it was years ago. I think this is due to the fact that mothers are better educated in nutrition these days and have a good basic knowledge of how to feed their offspring.

In anaemia the complexion is very pallid and the nails, the lips, the gums and the inner sides of the eye lids are similarly affected, the eyes glitter and the white parts are sky blue. The patient suffers from breathlessness, palpitations, fainting fits, indigestion, constipation, neuralgia and dropsy, also coldness of the extremities. Humming noises may be heard, spots and shadows may float before the eyes, the muscles may feel sore and there may be backache. In some cases the appetite is very capricious, and the patient may crave for particular foods.

Treatment

Constipation, if present, must be relieved by an aperient, and in my opinion one teaspoonful of black molasses three times daily cannot be beaten. It is an excellent laxative, whilst containing an abundance of iron and minerals. Iron of course is the great remedy for anaemia but this should always be given with vitamin C to absorb it. In my opinion 100 mg of iron daily and 500 mg of vitamin C are very useful. Whilst reliance is placed chiefly on the administration of iron and vitamin C, diet and hygenic measures must receive their due share of attention. Skimmed milk is very valuable, as are lamb and chicken, minced and reduced to a pulp, and flavoured with broth. Cod liver oil, if it can be digested, is to be recommended. Egg yolk, beaten up with a little water and flavoured with honey, is a valuable food, rich in iron. As the patient gains ground, solid, but not rich, animal food may be taken, and a good wholefood diet (described at the back of book) should be adopted. Iron and vitamin C should be taken daily in the quantities mentioned until all signs of anaemia have passed, and thereafter a daily intake of 50 mg iron and 500 mg vitamin C.

Secondary Anaemia

What has been said about the treatment of primary anaemia applies for the most part to anaemias that are the result of some other condition, whether it be haemorrhage, Bright's disease, cancer, chronic poisoning by such metals as lead, mercury, arsenic or copper, or disease of the organs which are concerned in the making of blood. However, there is one form of secondary anaemia which must be considered separately—the form known as pernicious anaemia. This type of anaemia was deemed fatal until 1926, when it was found to be treatable with large doses of raw liver. Then in 1948 vitamin B_{12} was isolated, and since then this type of anaemia has been relatively easy to treat.

Pernicious Anaemia

The cause is unknown. Sometimes it is ushered in by gastric and intestinal troubles, or by nervous shock or worry. More often, however, it comes on insidiously, and the first symptoms to attract attention are pallor, lassitude and muscular weakness. Breathlessness and fainting fits, with a tendency to palpitations then follow. The appetite fails, the mucous membranes of the eye and mouth become pale, the skin takes on a waxy or lemon tint, the muscles grow flabby, the temperature is often high but not considerably so, vomiting and diarrhoea are frequently present, and there is usually dropsy in the feet and ankles. Treatment should begin with bed rest and thereafter plenty of fresh air and sunshine and an abundant and nourishing whole-food diet. Injections of vitamin B_{12} are usually continued throughout life. A supplement of 100 mg iron and 500 mg vitamin C should be taken daily.

Thrush

The vagina is the name given to the passage leading from the exterior of the body to the womb. It can become inflamed, and sometimes the inflammation becomes acute and very stressful. In slight cases a discharge preceeds the menstrual flow—in severe cases it is constant. The seat of the infection can be anywhere along the genital tract in women—the uterus, cervix or vagina. Chronic inflammation can follow childbirth, or it can be due to gonorrhoea or simply to a lowering of health. The condition is not common in young children but if it does arise it is often due to a lowering of vitality, and general debility with lack of cleanliness. If the rash is persistent you should consult your doctor.

A distressing type of vaginal rash that, in the running of this Clinic, I very often meet, is thrush, caused by the administration of antibiotics. Sometimes when these are given for acute infection such as sore throat, bronchitis or whatever, they kill not only the bacilli responsible for the infection, but they also kill the friendly bacteria in the mucous membrane, and a very distressing itch is set up in the vagina region. At this stage the patient is in a very low state health-wise and the only treatment is a good nourishing diet coupled with a good multi-vitamin and multi-mineral, and also the addition of Superdophilus, which promotes the health of the mucous membrane; it can be obtained from this Clinic.

If vaginal discharge is due to erosion of the cervix (neck or the womb) or any other known cause, then of course this must be treated by the doctor. The general health of the patient should always be treated and a good diet, multi-vitamin and multi-mineral regime adopted. Live yoghurt is an excellent addition to the diet.

Cystitis

This condition is inflammation of the bladder caused by bacteria that live in the urine. In a healthy bladder they will not multiply, but if the bladder wall is weak or if a dirty catheter has been inserted then inflammation is set up. Hardening of the urethra, or enlargement of the prostate gland is a common cause of infection in elderly men. In women it is most commonly due to prolapse of the womb, which of course must be corrected. Sometimes a stone may be the cause due to its irritating action. The same symptoms, however, may be caused by bruising, and they can be treated in the same way.

The patient feels pain in the small of the back. The frequent urgency to pass water may be noticed and sometimes there is a bad smell and a white sediment in the urine. If the infection has become acute there may be a rise in temperature and shivering.

Treatment

At the first sign of an attack you should drink lots of water, and continue until you feel better. If you have a fever you should rest in bed until it passes. The application of hot water bottles to the lower abdomen may help to alleviate pain. When the acute stage has passed begin a gradual return to a good wholefood diet. You should avoid all refined carbohydrates—no white bread, no white sugar, use honey for sweetening. An acid-free diet is most important—this is described in detail in the chapter on arthritis (pages 68–74). One dessertspoon of cider vinegar in a glass of water and sweetened with honey three times a day produces wonderful results. Of course the addition of multi-vitamins and multi-minerals including zinc will result in optimum health. Many of my arthritis patients have been cystitis sufferers but, having spent a couple of months or thereabouts on their acid-free diet with cider vinegar, they joyfully report no more attacks of cystitis.

4

Skin Problems

Skin problems are many and varied and can have a variety of causes. Some skin eruptions are of nervous origin, others can be caused by local irritants, others again can be due to faulty diet such as too many refined carbohydrates or perhaps an inability of the liver and kidneys to function properly. The first line of action is to determine the cause of the eruption and once the cause is known there are various treatments at hand.

Nettle Rash

This is a name for a rash caused by an allergic reaction, usually to some kind of food. In this condition there is a sudden appearance of white or pink bumps of the skin, usually accompanied by a sensation of violent itching or burning. The commonest sites are the buttocks and the front and back of the chest. Sometimes one or two weals may appear and sometimes they may affect a considerable area of skin, and scratching or rubbing the skin tends to bring out weals during the course of nettle rash.

Digestive disturbances sometimes precede this condition, and very often there is a connection between the weals and eating fish, strawberries, eggs, meat or some kinds of cereal food. If the nettle rash keeps occurring a search should be made for some food to which the patient is sensitive and when found that food should be eliminated from the diet.

When nettle rash occurs, if the patient knows that he has taken something which has been responsible for the attack, the bowels should be cleansed by giving a good aperient such as senna pods or liquorice powder (see p. 25) and a fast of 24 hours on water only will help the cleansing process. A dusting powder containing zinc oxide will calm the rash, or a weak solution of warmed vinegar has a sedative effect.

Eczema

Eczema is an inflammation of the skin which may come into existence for no obvious reason. Like nettle rash, however, it is often caused by an allergic reaction to something in the diet.

Acute ezcema often appears first on the face. The skin becomes reddened, swollen and itchy and then hot and tense. Tiny blisters then appear, which sometimes become larger ones. Itching is a prominent symptom in most cases of eczema and when scratching the blisters rupture and pour out a clear sticky fluid. The disease may spread from the face or wherever it begins first to other parts of the body, and especially in children it may cover the whole body. If there is a lot of skin involved fever and loss of appetite may occur. While the skin is inflamed it is readily invaded by microbes which may cause pustules like impetigo or crops of boils.

The general treatment should include close scrutiny of the diet to try and fix responsibility, if possible, on a particular item, which can then be excluded from the diet. In severe cases a very light diet consisting of fresh fruit juices and vegetable juices, also water or barley water, should be given for the first 24 hours. Then a very gradual adding of fresh fruit and fresh vegetables. Alcohol, tea and coffee are not allowed. Then you can gradually return to a good wholefood diet.

Clothing next to the skin should be of cellular cotton with only sufficient bed and personal clothing to keep the patient comfortably warm. The bowels should be kept open. Calamine lotion is the usual local treatment.

Dermatitis

The term dermatitis covers several diseases, mostly related to allergy. It is an inflammation of the skin and may appear in any part of the body as blisters. Where it is caused by handling irritating substances it is known as contact dermatitis. Contact with oil or suds by those working in factories very often brings it on, and french polishers, gardeners and bakers often suffer from it. The dermatitis may last a long time after contact with the offending irritant has ceased, and it can cause depression.

Treatment consists of withdrawal from the offending irritant and the application of soothing ointments. Absolute cleanliness is essential. Sometimes too much sunshine can bring on what is known as sunshine dermatitis and here of course the treatment is to expose the skin to sunlight as little as possible, and apply a soothing lotion or ointment to the skin. It is especially important to recognize the cause of dermatitis in paraffin and tar workers, because if the irritation is allowed to operate for a long time a cancerous disease of the skin may be produced.

Poisonous substances in the blood may also be the cause of dermatitis. Often there is a clear connection between dermatitis and the administration of some drug. In this case you should stop taking the drug. Where there is heat and itching a sedative may be applied such as calomine lotion, a soothing dusting powder or an emollient like vaseline, lanolin, cold cream or zinc ointment.

Herpes or cold sores is another form of dermatitis occurring mainly in adults and it may be associated with some nervous disorder. In such cases a good wholefood diet should be adopted, and you should also take the following supplements daily until the condition clears:—

Zinc 45 mg
Vitamin C 2,000 mg
Vitamin E 400 international units.

The reduction of animal fat is important in these cases and of course no smoking.

Acne

This is a condition of the skin characterized by pimples and blackheads and they are collections of grease in the opening of the sweat glands, which are found especially on the face and neck. This is a difficult condition to treat but sometimes it can be helped by frequent washing with antiseptic soap. A good wholefood diet is very important containing plenty of green vegetables, raw or cooked.

Taking vitamin and mineral supplements not only helps the general overall health of the patient but also greatly increases the health of the skin. The following dosages should be taken:—

A good quality multi-vitamin daily
B complex 50 mg
Vitamin E 400 international units
Vitamin C 2,000 mg
Zinc 100 mg

Plenty of water should be drunk daily and it is important to avoid fried or fatty foods and white sugar. Smoking is taboo.

Acne Rosacea

This condition usually begins with flushing of the face due to such causes as menstruation or the menopause, pregnancy, defective circulation and excessive consumption of alcohol. As the condition becomes chronic the skin in the middle of the face becomes permanently red and pimples may arise. The skin of the nose becomes greatly thickened—this is known as rhinophyma and is mostly seen in habitual spirit drinkers. It is usually seen in middle or advanced life and is more common in men than in women.

Everything in the way of food that causes flushing should be avoided, particularly spicy foods. The bowels should be carefully regulated and the digestive organs maintained in good order. The treatment should follow the same lines as that advised for ordinary acne. In the more advanced stages, good results have been obtained by cauterization, electrolysis and x-rays.

Boils and Carbuncles

A boil may be described as an inflammatory swelling of the skin, originating either in one of its glands or in a hair follicle. The cause is a germ which finds entrance through some break in the surface of the skin; hence the frequency with which boils present themselves in places exposed to friction, for example on the neck where it is chafed by the collar. People who are troubled with boils frequently must be considered suffering from some predisposing condition of a constitutional kind, such as anaemia (see p. 32). Boils may also occur as a sequel of one of the infectious fevers, or perhaps such skin diseases as eczema, or in association with diabetes. One boil is very often quickly followed by a series of others. In many cases this may be the result of auto-infection—a boil when it has burst discharges germs which can easily be transmitted to other parts of the skin.

A boil usually starts with a little red pimple which is very tender. Soon it begins to harden and become inflamed. Usually the swelling enlarges and the surrounding tissues look 'angry'. After a while the swelling points and acquires a bright red blush on the surface. In a few days the boil bursts and a little matter is exuded. A little opening can be seen which leads right down to a greenish, yellow core, which in a day or two comes away and gives instant relief.

The local application of equal parts of set honey and black molasses is an excellent drawing and healing treatment. Spread the mixture on a little lint, cover with cotton wool and secure with micropore adhesive. (Micropore is a tape, obtainable from most chemists, which does not irritate the skin.) If the patient is debilitated he will need a good, wholesome diet, taking in plenty of green vegetables and fruit. A good multi-vitamin plus 500 mg calcium, 500 mg vitamin C and 50 mg iron daily.

A carbuncle is a large boil, usually found on the nape of the neck, but they can occur anywhere. Carbuncles are more deeply seated and are far more painful than boils. The swelling of a carbuncle may be as large as the palm of the hand, and the surface is dotted with several mattery points which break, releasing blood-stained matter. The duration of a carbuncle is much longer than a boil—it could last as long as two months. The patient feels ill and has shivering fits, fever and aching limbs. He should be given plenty of fluids and the same diet and vitamins as for boils. The lower bowels should be kept well regulated.

Dandruff

The cause is unknown but is probably due to some micro-organism. It is the cause of certain varieties of baldness and many skin erruptions, especially those affecting the chest, shoulders and arms. Patients infect themselves by scratching the scalp and then other parts of the body, or by combing the hair over bare shoulders.

In very young children it forms a greenish, scaly layer on the scalp, which should be bathed with water containing bicarbonate of soda, a teaspoonful to a pint. Then a little white vaseline should be rubbed in gently. This may be done daily after bathing.

In adults the scalp should be washed with the following:– 2 tablespoons of purified soft soap mixed with 2 tablespoons of methylated spirit, added to half a pint of warm water and used as a hair wash. Rub thoroughly into the scalp and roots of the hairs. Then dry with rough towels using considerable friction to the scalp. A sulphur ointment diluted with an equal part of vaseline should then be rubbed in gently, to separate the hair. The treatment should be carried out three or four times a week if possible. Use a stiff hair brush frequently, and wash the brush every week with a little soda or ammonia water.

An innumerable amount of skin erruptions owe their commencement to dandruff. A little greasy application, for example olive oil, should always be used after washing the scalp.

Baldness

Gradual hair loss occurs naturally in many people, and un-fortunately there is no known remedy for this kind of baldness. Onset is hereditary, and it may happen quite early in life. It is much more frequent in men than in women. Sudden dramatic hair loss is called alopecia aerata, and it can be the result of dandruff, anaemia, myxoedema, syphilis or nervous shock. After bad attacks of fevers the hair may fall out as the result of enfeeblement of the body, but with the return to health the hair will grow as before.

Treatment consists of absolute cleanliness. No hard brush or sharp comb should be used, as their irritation may aggravate the scalp. The head should be frequently washed, say once a week, preferably using a super fatted soap, or a whipped up egg as a shampoo. The hair should then be rinsed well and a final rinsing of half a cup cider vinegar added to one pint of cold water applied and left on. This promotes the acid-alkali balance in the scalp and gives a beautiful sheen to the hair. As in the case of disease attention must be paid to maintaining as high a standard of general health and healthy living as possible. You must not smoke, and you should adopt a wholefood diet in conjunction with taking the following vitamins and minerals every day:—

Silica 4 tabs
A good multivitamin
B Complex 100 mg
Vitamin C 1000 mg

Scabies (the Itch)

This is caused by a small insect which burrows into the skin and causes great irritation. In some cases intense rash and small abscess formation in the skin results. The commonest parts attacked are between the fingers and toes, but through scratching or by the clothes they may be transferred higher up the arms and legs or to any part of the body. The burrows may be seen as little streaks with a dark dot at one end which contains the insect. Itching is intense and is worse at night.

Treatment
The patient should give himself a thorough scrub in a hot bath with plain soap and water for half an hour, then rub himself well with sulphur ointment, put on clean night clothing and get into a fresh bed—clean sheets and blankets. The infected bed-clothing must be thoroughly boiled or otherwise disinfected, otherwise they re-infect the body. In the morning clean clothes should be worn. You should repeat the bath and application for four days. Gloves should be burned.

In any local forms of itching keep the parts clean and dry and investigate the cause.

5

Diseases of the Muscles and Nerves

Pains in the muscles can be debilitating, although there is a lot you can do to help yourself, without resorting to drugs and painkillers. In this chapter I also discuss heart disease and angina, which are becoming ever more prevalent.

Illnesses which result from inadequate diet can affect the nerves and the mind as well as the body, and I include here a section on diseases of the nerves, which often occur when the body is run down.

Strains

Overstretching of a muscle is described as a strain. There is pain and stiffness. The muscle should be rested, and massage and gentle movement will help. Hot or cold fomentations can also be used to relieve the pain. A fomentation is a compress or poultice, either warm and moist, or an ice bag or a flannel wrung out in ice-cold water. A fomentation can be applied to any part of the body, and alternate hot and cold compresses are very effective for promoting circulation and so relieving pain.

Violent stretching or a blow may rupture the muscle, in which case the limb should be placed in such a position as to put the muscle at rest. Sometimes the tendon of a muscle is displaced, causing pain and stiffness. In this a doctor will have to rectify the position and the limb will have to be rested completely for six or eight weeks. Sometimes, however, an operation is necessary.

Other muscular pains happen for a variety of reasons. Sometimes inflammation of a muscle can occur, and if the cause is a microbe an abscess may result. Muscular rheumatism is inflammation in the connective tissue mingled throughout a muscle. A painful spasm of a muscle is referred to as cramp, and pain in a muscle without signs of inflammation is spoken of as myalgia—it is usually due to rheumatism.

Disease of the muscles causes reduction in size and wasting. Disease of the nerve cells supplying the muscles is called neuritis, and this also results in wasting of the muscles. There may be a progressive muscular wasting involving all parts of the body, known as muscular paralysis. In all these conditions, the patient's general health is the first consideration. A good wholefood diet should be adopted and sometimes the taking of a potassium supplement brings about an improvement.

Muscular rheumatism (Fibrositis)

This is inflammation of the connective tissue in the muscles, which is widely distributed throughout the body. The inflamed tissue is first enlarged by an exudation of fluid so that it forms a swelling. When the swelling occurs it presses on nerves and may give rise to intense pain. Exposure to damp and cold should be avoided as much as possible. Fibrositis in certain regions of the body receives a special name. When it occurs in the lumbar region it is called lumbago. Sometimes it occurs in the intercostal muscles (the muscles between the ribs), and this is called pleurodynia. It is the commonest cause of stiff neck.

If the fibrositis is acute there is a great urgency to relieve pain and the most effective agents are heat or massage, or a combination of both. Heat may be applied in a variety of ways, such as a hot epsom salts bath, poultices, hot fomentations or hot water bottles. Massage should be gentle when done over tender spots. After the massage the patient should be encouraged to exercise the affected muscles. In severe cases you may have to resort to the use of aspirin for the relief of pain—but it should only be taken when the pain is bad, as it can cause bleeding of the stomach in some people, or stomach ulcers. The patient should be kept warm and should avoid draughts, and should wear warm underclothing. When improvement has occurred, rubbing with warm olive oil will improve the situation. A wholefood diet should be adopted and adhered to, and the taking of a good B complex and vitamin C daily, together with a good multi-vitamin, should help enormously.

Backache

The back is often the seat of an aching pain which may be very disabling. It can be caused by many things and affect different parts of the back. Often it accompanies a fever, and it is very marked in influenza. Sometimes a pain between the shoulders is common in stomach disorders, and in gall-stones the pain often strikes up the back of the right shoulder. In piles there may be a dull pain at the bottom of the spine. A dragging pain often occurs in women suffering from disorders of the womb. It may also be caused by mususe of the back muscles—bad posture or incorrect lifting positions.

The treatment of backache condition should be directed to the cause, but the application of heat usually produces some benefit, though it may be temporary. Rest in bed with a hot water bottle to the back and two B complex tablets with a hot drink often gives a lot of relief.

Massage is also effective, particularly with lumbago, where the pain is often severe. The patient should sit astride a chair and the painful part of his back kneaded with the thumbs, but pressure should not be sufficient to cause pain. The two thumbs are then placed on either side of the spine below the painful spot and the patient is directed to bend backwards and forwards and to turn his body round, first to one side and then to the other, these movements to be repeated several times. A surprising amount of relief will often be secured in this way.

There is a very painful condition of the spine known as a slipped disc, where absolute rest is essential on a rigid surface. A competent osteopath can put this right very quickly. It can be due to a number of causes and may occur again and again. If it does, you must avoid lifting any heavy weights, and sudden movements of the spine. Prevention is better than cure—this applies especially to this very painful condition.

Some backache is caused by weakness of the muscles used

when standing. The pain is chiefly felt in the small of the back and is much increased by exercise, and is always more severe when the patient is tired or in ill health. It is particularly liable to attack women who have had frequent pregnancies or who have nursed their babies too long. Sedentary habits are a predisposing cause. The trouble is relieved by rest in the recumbent position and by massage of the painful muscles. All causes of exhaustion should be avoided, the general health should carefully be attended to, and while moderate exercise is distinctly beneficial it should always be followed by a period of rest.

Pain may also be caused by injury to the coccyx, the curved bone in which the spinal column ends. This is not strictly a pain in the back but it may be considered here. One of the most frequent causes of this trouble is injury during labour, especially if forceps have to be used. Another is a sudden fall on a hard object—such as the stairs, or backwards onto a road or pavement—and any violent strain or injury can cause backache. Severe constipation and piles may also be responsible, while some cases are considered to be of a rheumatic or neuralgic character. However caused, the pain is usually considerable, and in some cases almost unbearable. If the trouble is caused by injury, hot fomentations and gentle massage with complete rest will soon give relief. In neglected cases and in those thought to be due to neuralgia and rheumatism the pain is prone to persist. General treatment consists in nutritious food, a change of air if possible, and the adoption of the Margaret Hills treatment for arthritis and rheumatism referred to in the chapter on arthritis. Care of the bowels is most important and special attention should be paid to the nervous system—stresses and strains should be avoided as much as possible.

In some cases backache is caused by disease in the spinal column, or in the spinal cord, or the membranes that cover it. These are serious conditions that must be treated medically. If the pain is high up in the back, between the shoulders, it may be an indication that there is something wrong with the digestion. If so it will probably be worse after taking food and there may be vomiting and pain in the pit of the stomach. Treatment for relief of the indigestion should be followed.

Pain due to kidney trouble is felt lower down the back, in the loins and may spread round to the abdomen and down to the groins. If the cause is stone in, or inflammation of, the kidney, pressure over the spot will cause tenderness; the bladder will be irritable, so that water has to be passed frequently, and the urine will also probably show some definite change from the normal. In healthy young women an aching pain in this region is sometimes caused by their taking too little fluid. As a result of this the urine is very concentrated and sets up irritation in the kidneys. The remedy is to drink more water or other liquid so that the solid substances in the urine may be kept in a state of solution.

In conclusion, another form of backache may be due to intestinal irregularity in the form of chronic constipation or of distension of the bowel with wind. In the former case the pain may be accompanied by irritation of the bowel set up by the hardening faeces. Treatment should be that adopted for constipation (see pages 24–25).

Cramp

This is an early sign of the exhaustion of nerve centres and should be a warning for rest. Writers, violinists, pianists, dancers and others who use the same muscles for long periods suffer from a spasm of the affected muscles, entirely preventing their use for some time. In writer's cramp the forefingers and thumb are most commonly affected—the pen may be twisted about in the grip or even thrown away by the spasm. In some forms the pen is so firmly gripped by the fingers it can only be removed with difficulty. Then a sense of uselessness and weakness follows, with peculiar sensations in the part, sometimes of numbness, and the skin may become shiny and red.

Treatment

Rest and change are two absolute essentials. In some cases of dancer's cramp a few days' rest and massage with warmed olive oil or Olbas oil will entirely relieve the condition, and a brisk rubbing before undertaking the dance should prevent cramp. In the other forms more prolonged rest is necessary and massage should be systematically carried out. The taking of vitamins A and D and calcium, iron and vitamin C should help to prevent recurrences.

Massage

Massage is an art which depends upon a knowledge of anatomy for its scientific application. But some massage is better than none, and good results can be obtained by carefully following the instructions now given. The process of massage combines various movements which are used singly or in combination. In most cases gentle force is all that is needed.

Most people rub up and down with equal pressure—this is not correct. Massage rubbing is a mixed stroking and kneading movement. All rubbing, stroking or other movements should always be directed upwards on the limbs and downwards on the head and neck, because this is the direction in which the nervous blood and lymph flow, and in all conditions calling for massage these two streams need stimulating and helping. Stroking or rubbing in the wrong direction retards rather than helps the current in its flow.

Stroking

Stroking is the movement by which all massage begins, and is called for especially in the course of acute inflammations or painful conditions of the skin and nerves. It may be performed with varying degrees of force and if the part is very tender only gentle stroking with the palms of the fingers can be borne. When the pain has subsided firmer stroking can be performed and the palm of the hand used, either flat as in rubbing or by grasping the limb between the fingers and thumbs. If the limb or part be large, the palm of one hand may be placed on one side and the other palm on the opposite side and both pushed towards the trunk either together or alternately. If the latter, one palm must begin its strokes just as the other ends.

Kneading

Kneading is the most useful of all movements for dispersing

chronic inflammations. After paralysis or wasting of muscles from long continued disease, or to prevent wasting from such causes, kneading is invaluable . It softens and makes supple a part of the body, just as kneading and working putty softens it. As the name indicates, the tissues are thoroughly manipulated. The only precautions are to avoid using so much force as to bruise the delicate tissues and always to do the kneading from below upwards. There are several ways of doing this:

- A piece of muscle may be picked up between the index finger and thumb and rolled between them five or six times, then the piece immediately above is taken and the process repeated until the whole muscle is treated.
- If the muscle is large it may be grasped between the fingers and the thumb, and the latter used to knead, roll and squeeze it against the fingers.
- The whole limb may be grasped with the thumbs in front and fingers behind and the tissues squeezed against the bones then relaxed and squeezed again. The whole limb from ankle to knee, say, should be gone over carefully from below upwards. The squeezing is done just as a wet sponge is squeezed, and the results can be very beneficial, as in this way the blood supply is encouraged and the vitality of the part increased.
- Again the limb may be grasped between the thumbs in front and the fingers behind, but with one hand higher than the other, now squeeze firmly, then roll the muscles with the hands as if wringing them.
- The last method consists in rolling the limb between the palms as if twiddling a stick or warming the hands when cold.

Friction

This is most useful in the treatment of long-term problem joints, and after sprains. It is really a deep firm stroking movement best performed with the tips of the fingers or with the thumbs. It helps to produce absorption of inflammatory products by breaking up the coagulated materials and by stimulating the circulation it helps in the process of repair.

Swimmer's cramp. This usually involves spasm of the arteries as well as the muscles, due to cold and exertion. The only treatment that can be applied is warmth and massage, also hot drinks.

Heat cramps. These are due to excessive loss of salt, mainly found in people working in extremely hot conditions such as factory foundries. The treatment consists of giving salt water to drink.

Night cramps. These come on during sleep. Suddenly there is an agonized feeling of pain in the back of the thigh or calf, or sometimes the toes. The muscles affected are gathered up into a hard painful mass, and this may last from a few seconds to a few hours. Usually the sharp pain disappears fairly quickly, leaving behind a dull ache. It is very common in arthritics—some of my patients have dreadful nights of cramp.

Treatment consists of grasping firmly and rubbing the affected part. Sometimes the application of cold water or stretching the limbs will help the immediate situation. If the patient can get out of bed a walk round helps tremendously. I give my patients calcium pantothenate and bonemeal and having spent approximately three weeks on this they report a lessening of cramp or no cramp at all. I also give a good multi-vitamin.

Other Muscular Problems

There are other, more serious diseases which can affect the muscles, and these include Parkinson's disease, Bell's palsy (facial paralysis), paraplegia and hemiplegia. Even where there is no cure it is important to attend to the patient's general health and hygiene, and give a good wholefood diet, with a multi-vitamin, B complex and vitamin C. Massage can also be helpful.

Heart disease

The heart is the most powerful muscle in the body. Disordered action of the heart sometimes occurs, called DAH, but this doesn't mean that there is anything organically wrong with the heart and should not be worried about.

Sometimes an acute infectious disease may be followed by shortness of breath on slight exertion, faintness, giddiness, palpitation, pain over the heart region and so on. Sometimes people with a nervous disposition may experience such symptoms, and in such cases a search should be made by the doctor for any source of bacterial toxaemia at the roots of the teeth, in the nose, in the tonsils and the appendix. However, in this book, we are mainly concerned with self help—what we can do to ward off such symptoms—and here again we come back to the regime of plenty of fresh air, exercise, and good wholesome food supplemented by a good multi-vitamin and B complex.

Heart disease can occur from acute rheumatism and this is a very serious condition. Here I speak with first hand experience—I developed it at 21 years of age. Perhaps you have read my first book, *Curing Arthritis the Drug-Free Way*, where I have referred to it. To begin with I got a very severe tonsillitis followed by rheumatic nodules on my legs, joint pains and soreness and a very enlarged heart. At that time I was a first year student nurse at St Stephen's Hospital, in London.

I was confined to bed for five months on complete rest—not allowed to wash or feed myself, and a Harley Street heart specialist called every other day to note my progress. When eventually I was allowed to get up and gradually wash and feed myself I was given the following advice: I should never cycle or dance again; I should never run uphill or upstairs; I should never have any children; I should never think of coming back to continue my nursing training—it would be too strenuous for my heart. That was very good advice and it is the advice I would give anybody today that would encounter the same situation. However, I did not take that advice. I was young and foolish, but fortunately for me my foolishness paid off and having disobeyed every advice I was given I seem to have come out on top. I cycled and danced at every available opportunity, I was accepted back at the hospital to finish my training and then I got married and had eight children.

I have since led a very busy life, bringing up those children and I also fostered one. Then when they were off my hands, I took a refresher course in nursing and nursed in the district and in factory surgeries for six years. At 57 years of age I opened a clinic here at my home in Coventry for arthritics. The clinic is very busy, and the results astounding. This is my third book—the other two—*Curing Arthritis the Drug-Free Way* and a companion diet book, *Curing Arthritis Cookbook*—are published by Sheldon Press and have been most successful. Nobody can say that I've sat back and taken life easy, and when I had to have a medical for obtaining an insurance on my life about 15 years ago my heart was in perfect condition. I often think how much I would have missed out on, had I taken the doctor's advice! It seems to me that sometimes the heart can make a full recovery if given the right conditions—good food, exercise, no over-exertion. I made a full recovery and I am so grateful—I am now 62 and still here to tell the tale.

Treatment

Do not worry about your heart condition, as this makes things worse and aggravates the condition. Do your best to live carefully, observing the rules of personal hygiene.

Constipation, indigestion and anaemia should be corrected. Smoking should be cut out but a little brandy now and again is a good tonic. Over-exertion should be avoided. A young person with heart trouble should choose an occupation which should not subject him to anything of this kind. Persons who are engaged in manual labour should live as near as possible to their place of employment, if they have to walk to work.

A patient suffering from heart trouble should take regular exercise if his employment is a sedentary one, keeping him indoors. Easy walking or games which do not put one out of breath are useful, as exercise flushes the muscles with nourishing blood and clears out waste products from them. If the patient is confined to bed, regular massage is a very good substitute.

A good wholesome diet should be taken, together with a good multi-vitamin, also 400 international units of vitamin E daily—

this strengthens the heart muscle and protects the artery walls. This vitamin is largely found in leafy, green vegetables, in wheatgerm and whole-grain foods. It acts as an anti-coagulant, keeping the blood running freely, thereby being extremely good in thrombosis. It is a wonderful medium in the healing of scars and for the promotion of healthy skin. People with high blood pressure should start with a small dosage—neither the required daily amount nor the toxic level is established, but the dosage is between 400 and 2,000 international units.

I have found that in treating my patients who suffer from any form of heart trouble, angina or high blood pressure this daily dosage of 400 international units of vitamin E, combined with 500 mg of lecithin helps enormously, and varicose veins have disappeared completely in many. The lecithin also prevents the formation of cholesterol in the blood vessels and is also a fat emulsifier. Those suffering from heart trouble of any description should be careful with their weight—many have a tendency to put on weight, but of course when this happens an extra strain is put on the heart so making matters worse.

Angina

Angina is very prevalent today. Intense pain is felt over the chest, accompanied by a feeling of constriction as though the chest was compressed in a vice. The pain may shoot through to the back and down the left arm and sometimes also down the right arm. The patient is frightened to breathe in case of sudden death, and stands motionless. The whole body is covered in a clammy sweat and the face is pale, the pulse is slow and feeble and the breathing short and hurried. As a rule the attack lasts a few minutes or even seconds, but may continue with varying intensity for much longer.

People suffering with angina are always under a doctor's guidance but they can do a lot to ward off attacks and help themselves. Treatment between attacks must be directed to avoiding any condition that is known to excite them. The diet should be simple, light and nutritious and the bowels kept in regular action. Rest after a meal is very important. Gentle exercise should be taken daily and if ordinary exercise is out of the question it should be replaced by a massage. The taking of vitamin E (400 international units) and lecithin (500 mg), referred to previously should be adhered to daily. Hot baths should always be avoided in any form of heart trouble.

Diseases of the Nerves

Disease of the nerves can be due to various factors such as lowered vitality due to faulty diet, strain, injury, stress, tension or deficiency of the B complex vitamins. On the other hand, the muscles can be diseased through strain or hyperacidity—as in the case of rheumatism—and mostly due to faulty diet. The cause should be ascertained and treatment carried out accordingly. In all cases a good, sensible, wholefood diet should be followed and exercise taken daily.

Sleeplessness

Insomnia arises from all kinds of illness, anxiety, pain, fatigue, especially from brain work, and in a large number of cases it is due to preventable causes, especially dietetic errors. Eating certain foods before retiring leads to flatulence and distension of the stomach, which presses upon the heart and causes great oppression. The sufferer must learn from experience which foods are responsible. Also taking coffee, tea or alcohol, and in some people smoking on going to bed excite the heart. Insufficiency of food and hunger, deficient bedclothing, cold feet, defective ventilation, too little exercise and absence of 'healthy' fatigue all contribute to sleeplessness.

Treatment is to avoid anything which is indigestible. Do not take a meal too late, but on the other hand do not go to bed hungry. Regulate the bowels and avoid constipation. If you are obliged to study at night take a brisk walk before going to bed. If over-fatigued a warm bath followed by a glass of hot milk, Ovaltine or Horlicks, or a little wine half an hour before retiring may induce sleep.

If the patient suffers from flatulence a glass of water as hot as you can bear, with half a teaspoon of bicarbonate of soda added taken in sips is useful just before going to bed. Peppermint water helps to relieve the condition—infuse fresh or dried mint in boiling water and drink warm.

Palpitations

This is a rapid, noticeable beating of the heart, and when due to heart or nervous disorders must be treated accordingly. Sufferers should like down and rest during an attack and avoid all excitement and exertion. When due to flatulence, a common cause, the accumulated wind in the stomach may be dispersed by taking sal volatile—20 drops in a little water—or five drops of peppermint essence on a lump of sugar, or by sipping very hot water. The application of fomentations and gentle massage to the front of the chest and pit of the stomach can be very helpful. Of course care should be exercised with diet. A high-fibre diet is excellent, and the bowels should be kept well open.

Hiccough

Hiccough is produced by innumerable causes, but chiefly by indiscretion in diet or by rapid eating, resulting in flatulence, or by taking hot or spiced foods. Dyspepsia, many nervous conditions, diseases of the bowel are also causes.

Treatment depends on the cause. Where this is unknown, sipping cold water is useful, or the application of a hot water bottle or massage with Olbas oil or warmed olive oil over the pit of the stomach may be beneficial.

Dizziness

In severe dizziness there is a sensation of whirling round or up and down. Alternatively the patient may appear himself to be steady while the objects around him are whirling, and sometimes the patient may fall to the ground or he may become sick and vomit.

A slight, more or less constant giddiness is common in neurasthenia, in chronic gastritis, in loss of elasticity of the arteries in elderly people (which is known as arteriosclerosis), and in those who use tea, coffee, alcohol or tobacco immoderately. It is also found in those whose vision is defective and who have a tendency to squint. People who have thickened arteries very often feel giddy when they look upwards and or sit or stand up quickly, for example in getting out of bed. A sudden severe attack of dizziness may be one of the symptoms of acute indigestion, when it is likely to be associated with headache, blurring of vision, sickness and vomiting.

The symptoms may be greatly relieved by vomiting—large amounts of tepid water will clear the stomach effectively. Another cause of sudden dizziness is epilepsy—perhaps preceding a fit, or as an attack of petit mal, which is the form of epilepsy in which the patient is not convulsed and the loss of consciousness is only momentary.

Dizziness may be connected with the ears—a plug of impacted wax, or even syringing may bring on giddiness or sickness. Disorders of the inner ear may bring on very frightening symptoms. There the giddiness is sudden and severe—the patient may fall and may lose consciousness for a moment, and there are noises in the head—hissing, blowing and banging and more or less deafness. Attacks such as these are likely to occur at longer or shorter intervals and meanwhile there may be a persistent slight giddiness.

Treatment depends on the cause in each case, but a lot can be done by the avoidance of smoking and excessive drinking of alcohol, tea, coffee. A good wholefood diet should be adhered to. A good vitamin/mineral supplement should be taken daily, together with 50 mg B complex, 50 mg iron and 1,000 mg vitamin C.

Nervous Breakdown

This is a common term for any emotional illness which makes it impossible for a person to cope with the stresses and strains of life. The person feels very tired, depressed and inadequate, and persistently anxious. This state very often leads to a stage when the person is no longer able to carry out his normal duties and can no longer be termed a responsible member of the community. There is great weakness and irritability.

Usually this condition is produced by over-fatigue, both mental and physical, worry, anxiety and by many exhausting diseases, among them influenza. In most cases it may be regarded as the wear and tear of life in a strenuous age. The most definite form is that which is brought about by shock to the nervous system. It can be from direct injury to the nerves or from fright or from horror at the sight of accidents to others.

The symptoms include pain and crawling sensations in the head and various parts of the body. In some cases there is a sense of pressure at the top of the head, and the patient may complain of tenderness or weakness of the spine. Another symptom, especially in women, is flatulence, and there may be dilation of the stomach and constipation, together with sinking or fainting feelings. Very often the pulse is fast. Mental symptoms may occur—for example the patient may magnify small incidents, especially those connected with his or her health. Generally it may be said that the patient worries unnecessarily, and loses all self-confidence.

The mildest form of breakdown is that which is often met with at the end of a year's work. The person is mentally and physically exhausted, work becomes an effort, there is lack of concentration and mere trifles are magnified out of all proportion to their importance. In this form of debility the annual holiday may be the answer.

Treatment

In serious cases nothing short of a rest-cure is efficacious. It will probably have to be maintained for at least two months, and in some cases much longer. The patient should go to a nursing home, and be protected from everything that would worry and disturb him. He should have plenty of rest, and take regular exercise.

He should have a good wholefood diet together with the supplement recommended for dizziness. The bowels should be carefully regulated.

6
Fevers

The commonest contagious fevers are measles, scarlet fever, whooping cough, mumps, chicken pox and german measles. Each of these diseases has a period during which the disease is developed in the body, usually without any visible sign, and this is called the incubation period. Then the disease shows itself by certain symptoms, which may either be sudden or gradual—this is called the onset. Then nearly all develop a rash which is seen first on some definite area of the body. The progress of the disease is marked by stages which eventually end in convalescence. During this time however, the patient is for a longer or shorter period still contagious, or infectious to others through any kind of contact. Anyone who has been in contact with such a patient, before being considered free of acquiring the disease, should undergo a period of quarantine.

In all kinds of fevers bed rest is most important. The rise in temperature indicates that the body is endeavouring to get rid of the toxic wastes that have accumulated therein. In this process the body needs help, not through drugs or antibiotics, but through encouraging perspiration—hot drinks of cider vinegar and honey should be given frequently, or hot lemon juice or herbal teas, particularly peppermint tea. The cause of high temperatures in children should always be ascertained—the doctor should be called in. The patient should stay in bed until the temperature is normal.

How to recognise its signs and symptoms

- Fever may occur suddenly with a rise of temperature, up to 106°F, 41°C
  The temperature should be taken in the armpit or mouth. A slightly higher temperature is obtained in the mouth than in the armpit.

- A rigor or chilly sensation—in children it is often ushered in by convulsions
- The face is flushed
- Increased frequency of pulse and respiration
- The throat is dry, tongue white coated. In some cases there is dry mucous on lips and teeth
- Loss of appetite
- Hot, dry, pungent skin
- Eyes bright and glistening or sometimes watery
- Constipation and scanty amount of urine
- Feeling of great lassitude and loss of strength
- Considerable restlessness

Where the patient is exceedingly ill the character of the fever changes.

- The pulse becomes weak and irregular. Respiration is shallow.
- Patient becomes delirious, often muttering. The eyes may be half closed or bright and staring. Tongue may be dry, often cracking.
- Sometimes the patient may pick at the bedclothes, or try in a feeble way to catch imaginary objects in the air, or see objects on the wall.
- The skin tends to be very clammy. This latter condition is more common in those who have suffered much ill health or whose health has broken down through prolonged illness, starvation or weak constitution.

Measles

The period of incubation is 8 to 12 days. Onset in very young children may be by a convulsion or shivering fit. In older persons the temperature may rise to 104°F, 40°C. Other symptoms are running eyes and nose, sneezing, wheezy cough or hoarseness. This stage lasts 3 to 4 days.

On the fourth day a rash appears, consisting of dull, red, minute, slightly raised points. It is first seen behind the ears, on the temples and at the hair line, and the whole body is covered with rash in 24 hours. Usually the rash begins to fade on the third day. When the rash appears the fever may rise higher, but it should soon fall. If it continues high after the rash has disappeared, it is due to some complication; either bronchitis, pneumonia or earache and you should call the doctor. After measles, children must be kept away from school for three weeks after the rash disappears. The skin and nasal and eye discharges are all very infectious.

In fever connected with measles the patient should be isolated in a well-ventilated, darkened room, protecting the eyes from sunlight. Put the child to bed and avoid chills. Give a fluid diet and keep the bowels regular. During convalescence keep the child warm.

Scarlet Fever

The incubation period is 1 to 3 days. The symptoms of onset are sudden fever, sore throat, vomiting and the glands in the neck under the ears are swollen and tender. The rash appears about 24 hours after onset. It is bright red, very diffusely spread all over the body, and is uniform, not patchy. First it is seen on the neck and upper part of the chest, then in front and behind the ears, and then spread all over the body. The face is flushed but has no rash, and around the mouth and skin is markedly pale. The skin is hot and dry, and the tongue has a white fur on it, showing red raised points. The throat is very red and looks swollen and tender. The rash lasts from one to three days. The fever falls gradually from 104°F, 40°C, or less to normal. Complications like ear disease and inflammation of the kidneys, abscess in the neck and joint troubles will have to be watched for. The skin, nasal discharge and sputum are very infectious.

The treatment consists of isolation in bed in a suitable room, well ventilated. Diet during fever should always consist of fluids only and as the temperature abates a light nourishing diet should be adopted and from then onwards as the patient recovers the wholefood diet should be adopted and adhered to.

Bright's Disease

Bright's disease is an inflammation of the kidneys which sometimes occurs as a complication of scarlet fever. It can also be caused by exposure to cold, especially after muscular exertion which put some strain upon the kidneys and so renders them liable to chill. But this disease may also occur as a complication of various other diseases, or of pregnancy or it may be set up by alcoholic excess or by the action of certain irritant drugs. The disease usually begins with shivering fits and a rise of temperature accompanied by pain in the loins, nausea and vomiting. Other common symptoms are headache, a furred tongue and constipation.

Medical diagnosis is necessary and the usual medical treatment today is an antibiotic. This I don't agree with. I have treated acute kidney disease in my daughter Christine very successfully by the following method. Instead of giving the prescribed antibiotic I fasted her on fresh orange juice only—two ounces every two hours for three days to clear the system, then grapes only for two days. At the end of those five days she returned to the doctor with a second sample of urine which showed that she was absolutely clear. He thought she had taken the antibiotic he had prescribed for her five days previously and was very pleased to tell her that it had worked. She did not tell him that she hadn't taken it—she was scared in case he was annoyed. Her kidney infection did not return for approximately 25 years, when we used the same treatment and again all was well.

That incident when Christine was eleven years old gave me tremendous confidence in natural treatment, and since then in every situation in the family I have used natural treatment and got wonderful results, especially with eczema, pneumonia, acne and bronchial asthma. As I have said before, the results I am getting through treating arthritis the natural way are astounding, and of course it was with natural treatment I cleared my own arthritis 25 years ago.

Whooping Cough

Whooping cough is largely a disease of childhood, and incubation takes about eight days. The onset is insidious and begins with a troublesome cough, which is worse at night. Then there is fever, with restlessness and sneezing, getting worse and worse every evening. This lasts a few days, then the first stage of the disease begins.

There are three stages; catarrhal, spasmodic and declining. The catarrhal stage lasts 10 days as a rule, and may be known by the foregoing symptoms developing into an acute bronchitis or the cough becoming more hard, dry and troublesome with a little fever (100°F, 38°C), headache and malaise.

Towards the end of the second week the spasmodic stage begins. The cough becomes longer and louder, and more exhausting. It appears to come on in the form of attacks which are worse towards evening, and the intervals between the attacks are now more definite. After two or three days the characteristic whoop appears. The child's face becomes red, he gives a series of short, quick, forcible expiratory efforts, then the breath drawn in quickly with a whoop or whistling sound. Three or four such whoops occur, then the child is sick, or it brings up a lot of thick white phlegm through its mouth or nose. The child soon knows of approaching attacks, and dreads them. Attacks leave the child quite exhausted and often bleeding from the nose and lungs. The third stage, subsiding spasm and attacks, is reached in four to six weeks, but a cough with loose phlegm may last for a long time. The disease appears singly or in epidemics, and the infection seems greatest during the first week of illness, but lasts a month after commencement of the whoop. The patient should avoid contact with other children for approximately five weeks.

Treatment

The patient should be kept in bed until the temperature is normal. Plenty of rest, warmth, fresh air, and light nourishment should be given frequently in small quantities. During the catarrhal stage I have found nothing to equal the honey and onion cough mixture given for bronchitis (see p. 7).

During convalescence change of air and an iron tonic is advisable. Whooping cough immunization has proved very effective in warding off or lessening the symptoms and shortening the normal course of the disease.

Mumps

This is an infectious disease which may rapidly spread through a household of young children. There is usually fever, but rise of temperature is generally slight, and does not last long. The child is indisposed, peevish and somewhat pale. There is a swelling just below the ear and jaw, on one or both sides. Chewing and swallowing are painful, and the child does not feel like talking or running about. One side may be affected, then the other.

Treatment is for normal infectious fever. Isolation in a warm, well-ventilated room, a fluid diet and a good laxative will prove beneficial. If there is a lot of pain gentle massage with Olbas oil, or hot flannels sprinkled with Olbas oil and applied to the side of the face, may prove beneficial. The attack lasts five or six days and may then involve the opposite side. The child should not return to school for one month.

Chicken Pox

In this condition the incubation period is 10 to 15 days. The onset is gradual with slight headache, lassitude or chill with slight fever. In a few hours the rash appears first upon the back and chest or upon the face and forehead. It appears as rose-coloured spots. In approximately 24 hours these become blisters, which are small but increase in size and gradually become turbid. On the second day they are large in size and form matter, and usually they burst or dry up and form scabs. The patient may feel extremely ill, but usually the disease is mild.

Treatment consists of isolation until every trace of peeling has ceased. Careful nursing and the avoidance of chills and too early exposure are vital. The child should be prevented from scratching the pustules especially on the face, as pockmarks may remain. Calamine lotion may relieve the itching.

German Measles

The incubation period is 10 to 12 days. There is aching of the limbs, slight headache and giddiness, sometimes a chill and sore throat. Then the rash appears. In many cases the rash may be the first sign of the disease and is accompanied by fever. It begins in the face and in 24 hours has covered the body. It consists of slightly raised spots of a pinkish colour. It is patchy, more coarse than the rash of measles, and it usually persists 3 to 4 days and then slight peeling occurs. The glands at the back of the neck are swollen and tender.

The treatment consists of isolation for approximately 10 days and general nursing care as for the other fevers.

7

Arthritis

The word arthritis means inflammation of a joint or joints. There are two chief types; rheumatoid and osteo-arthritis.

I have written two books on this subject. The first, *Curing Arthritis—The Drug-Free Way* has become a bestseller, and the companion volume, *Curing Arthritis Cookbook* has recently been published. So much can be said about this subject, that I feel to understand the disease properly the reader would be well advised to purchase *Curing Arthritis—The Drug-Free Way*, published by Sheldon Press and on sale at most good bookshops and available from my clinic. The second book is a book of acid-free recipes specially compiled for the arthritic—diet is a most important factor.

I run a very busy clinic here in Coventry, specializing in arthritis and its associated diseases, called the Margaret Hills Clinic, and I have found that the cause of this painful disease is too much uric acid in the body. In my opinion this applies to both osteo- and rheumatoid arthritis. The treatment is simple and sensible—remove the cause and build up the patient's health.

I can relate so well to my suffering patients because from the time I was 21 years of age until I was 36 I suffered with both osteo- and rheumatoid arthritis. In those days phenylbutozone was the 'wonder drug' of the day—it has since been banned because of its dangerous side effects. Fortunately, I realized the implications of taking it, so for the excruciating pain I stuck with aspirin, although this too can cause bleeding of the stomach. I was totally crippled—I had it in every joint of my body and every movement was pain. It is said that 'necessity is the mother of invention' and it was certainly so in my case—I explored every avenue to get back to health, as I had six young children to bring up and no money to pay any help.

Being a State Registered Nurse helped a lot—it certainly helped me to decide that drugs were not the answer, so I turned

68

to alternatives. I tried many so-called cures until I hit on the 'combined treatment' that rid me of all signs of arthritis in twelve months. This treatment is the one I practise today in my clinic, and the results are astounding, even with patients who write in and adopt the treatment by post. The hundreds of letters I hold from people throughout the United Kingdom and abroad are testimonials to the excellent results produced. The clinic has been featured on radio and television throughout Britain in conjunction with my books.

If the reader has arthritis, take heart—you really don't have to 'learn to live with it', and in my opinion the drugs given for it will do more harm than good. Adopt the following natural treatment and feel yourself getting better, feeling stronger, more positive, more energetic day by day. Recovery is slow, but worth waiting for. You will have your set-backs—which I call flare ups—as you go through the treatment. These are a natural attempt by the body to throw the acids off, which produce inflammations where perhaps you haven't had them before, but they will pass, and you will feel so much better after you've had one than before. Give yourself time, be patient, be positive and above all don't give up—the results in the long run are well worth waiting for. I could have given up so many times, but I knew the alternative was drugs, which I feared, so I soon started to think straight again.

The following is the treatment programme I give to my patients. It consists of acid-removing treatment, an acid-free diet and high-quality supplements of vitamins, mineral, trace elements and protein. The reasoning behind this programme is, firstly, that arthritis is due to too much acid in the body, so that acid has to be removed—hence the acid-removing treatment. Secondly, it is most important not to allow offending acids back into the body during the acid-removing programme, and thirdly a good health-building programme is imperative to help the return to health. Because the arthritic is an ill person, those few pains and aches that you get now have a nasty way of confining you to a wheel chair in a few years.

Most arthritics are anaemic—sometimes due to drugs, sometimes due to the stress of pain. They suffer from cramp, pins and needles, depression, headaches, migraine, stomach ulcers, diverticulitis—all sorts of conditions, either drug induced or otherwise. They need the protein, vitamins and minerals so much, and benefit so much from them that sometimes if the post is late and they are without them for a day they are on the phone panicking. Every arthritic suffers in the same way to a greater or lesser degree. So they all start with the following basic treatment.

Treatment for the Relief of Arthritis

Acid-Removing Treatment

You will need

Clear or set honey	from
Cider vinegar	health food
Crude black molasses	stores
Epsom salts baths	from Boots

Dissolve one teaspoon of clear or set honey in a tumber of hot water. Add to this one dessertspoon of cider vinegar. Take three times daily. Take one teaspoon of black molasses three times daily. Black molasses is a laxative—start with one teaspoon daily and gradually build up.

Epsom Salts Baths. Dissolve one pound of epsom salts in a bath of comfortably hot water. Do not add soap or bath cubes. Keeping the water hot, soak for 10–15 minutes. Dry quickly and get straight into a warm bed. This bath may be taken three times weekly only as it tends to be weakening. People with any form of heart trouble should be careful not to have the water too hot. A good restful night's sleep is achieved.

Hand Baths and Feet Baths. Dissolve one teacupful of epsom salts in a bowl of water as hot as you can bear. Soak and exercise hands, wrists and fingers for 10–15 minutes. Dry hands and wrap in towel for five minutes for pores to close. Keeping the water hot, repeat on feet. These baths are excellent for the relief of pain in hands and feet.

The Acid-Free Diet

Any foods not mentioned are permitted in moderation.

Cereals	If eaten whole and in moderation, cereals are excellent. These include wheat, rye, barley, oats, millet, maize or brown rice, and of course 100% wholemeal bread.
Eggs	Three or four eggs a week is sufficient, because of the high cholesterol content.
Vegetables	Vegetables are a daily must. Eat them fresh and uncooked as far as possible.
Fruits	Eat apples, peaches, pears, bananas, apricots, melons, but avoid all citrus fruits such as oranges, lemons, grapefruit, mandarins, tangerines, and plums, pineapples, tomatoes, strawberries—in fact any fruit that is acid. A good rule of thumb to determine whether a fruit is acid is if your mouth waters when you think of it, it is acid—forget it.
Nuts and seeds	Taken daily these will improve your health. Avoid salted nuts.
Salt	Use only sea salt or biochemical salt, and then only in cooking.
Dairy foods	Do not use butter—use only vegetable margarines. Use dried or skimmed milk. Never use cream. In the cheese range, only cottage cheese is permitted.
White meats	Chicken, turkey, veal, rabbit, and duck occasionally, are excellent, also lamb.
Fish	White fish is an excellent source of protein and iodine, and should be eaten three or four times weekly. It may be prepared in any way except fried.

Red meats	Beef or pork, or any derivatives of these meats—corned beef, beef or pork paté, ham, bacon, sausages, pork pie, etc., should not be eaten.
Organ Meats	Lamb's liver, heart and brains are very good—but avoid kidneys.
White sugar	Not to be taken. Use honey for sweetness. No chocolate.
White bread	Not to be taken. All cakes and pastries made from white flour should be avoided.
Sauces and gravies	Sauces and gravies are permissible, using dried or skimmed milk where necessary.
Pickles and spices	All should be avoided as much as possible.
Drinks	Drink water in abundance—it is a wonderful body cleanser and of course it is a good source of minerals. Apple juice is also very good and any vegetable or fruit juices made in your blender, excluding citrus fruits. Avoid all short drinks and table wines. Weak tea and decaffeinated coffee is permissible.

Replacing Lacking Bodily Nutrients

The arthritic invariably suffers from iron deficiency, pins and needles, cramp, frayed nerves, depression, pain and a general depletion of bodily nutrients. It is imperative that these nutrients be replaced in the body to enable it to return to a state of health. These nutrients are available on application direct to the Margaret Hills Clinic.

CAUTION. This diet must not be adopted without taking the following nutrients which supply to the body the vital vitamins, minerals, and trace elements that are lost when acid foods are withdrawn. You will also need to replace protein with my protein formula.

The following is a list of the vitamins and minerals that I have found are invariably lacking in the arthritic, and when these are

72

supplied to the body a feeling of well-being is felt that has not been experienced for years. These vitamins are completely free of additives and colourings and made specially for the Margaret Hills Clinic, each daily intake consisting of:

Vitamin A	4,000 International Units
B Complex	50 mg
Vitamin C	500 mg
Vitamin D	400 International Units
Vitamin E	400 International Units
Calcium Pantothenate	500 mg
Bonemeal	900 mg
Kelp	500 mg
Selenium	100 mcg
Iron Orotate	50 mg
Alfalfa	500 mg

Sometimes, in fact more often than not, this has extremely good results, but as the patient progresses he may need more than the basic. For instance, if cramp is persistent extra calcium may be necessary, or if there is persistent numbness or pins and needles I have found that extra vitamin E with calcium produces excellent results. Sometimes there is persistent anaemia, and here natural iron and vitamin C is the answer. Many of my patients have very sleepless nights, very often due to pain, upset nerves or emotional stress, and all these conditions can be treated naturally, without the use of drugs and so much more effectively. Later on in this book you will find the effects that the various vitamins, minerals, trace elements and protein have on the body, and you will realize how necessary these nutrients are to the recovery of the sufferer.

In rheumatoid arthritis the soft parts of a joint become thickened, the cartilages, tendons and muscles waste away and the bone becomes thin, brittle and porous. In osteo-arthritis the cartilages and bones of a joint become enlarged, the bones become grooved and outgrowths are formed. In my opinion the cause of both of these conditions is too much acid in the body, and the inflammations are set up by poisons produced by germs, that, in a state of good health could not multiply and produce the pain and deformities that exist in both these conditions. Exposure to cold and damp, prolonged worry and overwork appear also to be contributing factors.

Acute arthritis deformans affects many joints at the same time and is accompanied, as a rule, by fever. In the chronic type of the disease the hands are usually attacked first, then the knees and feet and lastly, in very bad cases, nearly all the other joints of the body. In acute cases the inflamed joints must have complete rest, and the pain may be relieved by hot fomentation or hot epsom salts baths. It is important that as soon as the joints cease to be painful gentle movements should begin to be practised, and these must be continued perseveringly when the disease has passed into the chronic stage to prevent or lessen deformity. To this end light massage of the joints and neighbouring muscles is of great importance, and benefit may be derived from hot air baths. In many cases warm mineral baths are beneficial. The diet must be good, wholesome and acid-free as directed earlier. The acid-removing treatment should be adopted, and the vitamins and minerals listed in the Margaret Hills Formula—together with the Margaret Hills Protein daily.

8

Natural First Aid

Natural remedies are also useful for minor troubles and emergencies which arise in the home every day.

Bed Sores

In the nursing of the sick, especially if the patient is very aged and infirm or is affected by paralysis, it is often difficult to prevent bed sores. Patients who are compelled to use the bed pan or the urinal, and most of all those paralysed patients whose motions and urine pass involuntarily, are particularly liable to develop this trouble.

Cleanliness is of the utmost importance in all such cases. The draw sheet should be kept free of creases and changed as often as it becomes damp or soiled. Whenever possible the posture should be frequently changed so as to vary the pressure. Water and air beds and cushions should be used in all cases in which there is any danger of the occurrence of bed sores, but it will still be necessary to observe most scrupulously the precautions mentioned above. In addition, all the parts subject to pressure, after being washed and throughly dried, should be rubbed gently with some eau-de-cologne or methylated spirit until this has quite dried in, and should then be dusted with a starch and oxide of zinc powder.

While carefully carrying out all these preventive measures, the nurse must always be on the watch for the first indications of bed sores. As soon as any signs of a sore appears the part should be cleansed two or three times daily, dried thoroughly and covered with a small piece of lint smeared with zinc ointment or with vaseline. Over this, to protect the sore from pressure, should be placed a thick pad of cotton wool, with a hole cut in the centre rather larger than the piece of skin to be protected. This may be kept in place with micropore adhesive, or with a few turns of a bandage. Sometimes a compress of boric lint, wet with hot water, may be very beneficial. If the surface is raw it should be dressed two or three times a day, and some tincture of benzoin or zinc ointment applied.

Burns and scalds

The distinction between burns and scalds is simply that the latter are caused by moist heat such as steam, and the former by dry heat—the injuries produced are the same. Burning is a very common accident and many cases could be prevented by the knowledge and avoidance of certain risks. Young children should never be left alone in a room with an open fireplace or a stove, unless there is an efficient fire guard. Special care must be taken to keep clothing from naked lights of any sort. Many children have been burnt from standing in front of a fire in a nightdress. The delicacy of a young child's skin is such that serious burning may be caused by applying an overhot poultice, and hot water bottles should always be covered, and should be placed so that it does not touch any part of the body.

A burn of any severity is likely to be associated with the condition known as shock. It is important to remember that when this is so there may be no complaint of pain. It is sometimes assumed that a child who lies quiet and still cannot have suffered so much as might be expected. But the absence of crying has really grave significance. Children are much more likely to be affected in this way than are adults. Burns of the trunk are more likely to be attended with shock than those of the limbs, and large superficial burns rather than deep burns of a smaller surface.

In burns of any severity a doctor should always be summoned. In the meantime shock may be treated by putting the patient to bed and placing hot water bottles near him. Stimulants should be given freely—spirits of sal volatile in water, tea or coffee. Putting a child in a warm bath has at once the effect of relieving shock and of permitting easier removal of the clothing.

Great gentleness should be exercised in taking away clothing from the burnt surface, and if in spite of thorough soaking, it still adheres, it is better to cut round the adherent piece. Where there is broken skin greasy applications should not be made. The reason for this is that they may make the subsequent cleansing of the burn much more difficult, so that septic contamination may result.

The aim in all burns is to keep them free from infection. Where however there is merely reddening of the skin, zinc ointment, vaseline, cold cream or olive oil may be applied. Boracic acid powder or oxide of zinc are also very useful. Bicarbonate of soda is a good remedy when made into a thick paste with a little water and spread on thickly.

Large blisters should be pricked with a sterile needle, and the burns then covered with lint lightly wrung out of warm boracic solution. A limb with a burn may be immersed in a basin of water to which a tablespoon or boracic acid powder has been added. When a burn has not gone beyond the stage of blistering, there is unlikely to be scarring, but in deeper burns scarring will follow.

Earache

Put a drop of almond or olive oil into the ear, and then apply warmth.

Food poisoning

Most cases of food poisoning are due to a bacteria called salmonella. There are other causes but this is the most common. The salmonella bacillus may be present in canned or fresh food. Symptoms due to eating contaminated tinned food begin shortly after the food is consumed and suddenly there is vomiting, diarrhoea, abdominal pain, cramps in the limbs and some fever. Poisoning from fresh foods produces less abrupt symptoms that are less severe as a rule but last longer.

Vomiting and diarrhoea are usually sufficiently severe to clear the bowel, but this may be helped along by giving large amounts of tepid, boiled water, a dose of salts or castor oil. The patient must be kept lying down and must be kept warm. A hot water bottle helps the pain and cramps in the stomach.

In the course of bringing up my family of eight children I have, from time to time, encountered symptoms of food poisoning. My treatment consisted of the following which worked every time. To a small glass of tepid water I added 2 teaspoons of cider vinegar, and gave this to the patient to sip, this usually produced severe vomiting, and the patient continued to sip the cider vinegar mixture between bouts of vomiting, until in a very short time the stomach was emptied. No food was given for 24 hours but plenty of warm, boiled water, to which was added 2 teaspoons of cider vinegar. In this way a return to good health is invariably achieved and a feeling of extreme well-being.

Allergies can also produce food poisoning—see p. 37.

Headache

Give half a teaspoon of sal volatile in water. A mustard plaster to the nape of the neck and cold applications to the forehead are very beneficial.

Heartburn

Half a teaspoonful of bicarbonate of soda or magnesia in water will usually relieve the symptoms. Avoid greasy food and pastry.

Insect bites

Bathe with solution of ammonia, or bicarbonate of soda. Bites are sometimes prevented by spraying cuffs and tights with compound tincture of lavender and dabbing exposed parts with same. Mosquito bites are prevented by dabbing exposed parts with solution of epsom salts.

Itching

Put 1 heaped teaspoonful of bicarbonate of soda to 1 pint water as hot as you can bear, and sponge or bathe. Apply zinc ointment or zinc dusting powder.

Migraine Headaches

The cause is often hereditary. A gouty or rheumatic tendency, eye defects, short sight and squint, indigestion, chronic Bright's disease and a sluggish liver are common causes. Attacks may be brought on by excitement, fatigue, over-exertion, bad lights to work or read by, over-eating or want of sleep. They may occur at regular intervals of every two or three weeks.

Signs are peculiar—zig-zag lines or spots may be seen. This is followed by severe headache, perhaps beginning in a localized spot about the eye or temple. It then spreads gradually, usually over one side only, but both sides of the head may become affected. Vomiting or retching is common. The head is hot, blindness may persist during the attack. There is no fever but the pain is intense.

Treatment consists of avoiding or curing the cause of attack. Attention to bowels and feeding is most important. Have the eyes examined. If the sufferer is anaemic give suitable treatment with iron and vitamin C. A cup of hot coffee sometimes brings relief during the attack. Rest in a darkened room providing complete quietness is a must. Gentle massage by stroking the temple sometimes proves beneficial.

Sprains

If the sprain is severe it is difficult to exclude the possibility of fracture, so you should see your doctor at once.

If it is a simple sprain rest the part. If it is a lower limb keep it elevated, if the arm is affected put it in a sling. Applications of muslin soaked in cold water and vinegar are soothing. When the acute symptoms have subsided gentle massage and gentle moving of the joint will be beneficial, and an elastic bandage will give support.

Sting

Extract sting, then apply weak solution of household ammonia or sal volatile or solution of bicarbonate of soda. If there is severe inflammation or general illness a doctor must be called.

Stomach-ache

Various remedies can be beneficial. The following are all effective; half a teaspoon bicarbonate soda in water; bismuth and soda; peppermint water; five drops of essence of cinnamon or spirit of camphor on sugar; a hot water bottle or hot foment-ations applied to the pit of the stomach. In infants give sips of warm water and apply a warm flannel to the abdomen. Make sure feet are kept warm. If the stomach-ache is not speedily relieved, consult a doctor.

Toothache

Put cotton wool soaked in clove oil or spirit of camphor into the cavity of the tooth. Dry the gum and paint it with tincture of iodine. Apply a hot water bottle or bread poultice to the cheek.

9

The Value of Supplements

Practically everybody today needs to take supplements for the promotion and maintenance of good health. So many people today are over-fed but in fact under-nourished, because fruit and vegetables are very seldom eaten straight from the garden, the vitamins and minerals they contain are virtually destroyed through storing, chopping and cooking before they reach our tables.

Take, for example, vitamin C. Oranges are full of it until you peel them—in segmenting them and exposing the flesh to the air a lot of the vitamin C is lost. If they are chopped or blended, still more is lost, and the longer they are then kept, either in a fridge or out of it, the more vitamin C you lose, until eventually the amount of the vitamin consumed is minimal. Boiling vegetables is another example—the longer you boil the more vitamins are destroyed, until eventually the water contains more vitamins than the portion of green vegetables on your plate. Approximately 70 per cent of vitamins is removed from the whole grain when it is milled to produce white flour, and this is the reason that white bread and cakes made with white flour are not to be recommended—they are not bad for you but they certainly won't do you any good.

Bearing all this in mind we should resolve to keep our food as simple and as near to natural as possible. But even though we try and do this we can't win, because those good-looking vegetables and fruit have been grown for quantity and not quality, and they have been sprayed with chemicals and fertilizers, so to make sure of optimum health, vitamin and mineral supplements every day is the answer. Once you've started to take them the feeling of well-being is very evident—it is amazing the difference they make to your whole outlook. Digestion, elimination, nerves and circulation all benefit, but of course you must take the correct supplements for your body—it is no good taking vitamin E, for example, just because your next door neighbour takes it. A good basic knowledge of the individual vitamins is therefore essential, and if you are unsure you should see a specialist in this field.

We all know if we're not feeling well, and most of us know why. What we don't know is how to put it right. In the following pages I will endeavour to enumerate as far as possible the benefits derived from taking various supplements.

Vitamins—What are They?

Vitamins are food elements which are essential to growth and health, because of their importance to life. The word 'vitamin' comes from *vita*, which is Latin for 'life'.

Vitamin A

The first of them, vitamin A, is vital for healthy growth. It is found in green leaves and in milk, cream and butter, yolk of egg, fish oils and peanut oil. The deficiency of this substance in the diet of children used to cause rickets. Vitamin A is fat-soluble, which means that it needs fats as well as minerals to be properly absorbed by the body. It can be stored in the body and need not be taken daily.

It is measured in International Units—10,000 units daily is the recommended dosage. Its beneficial effects on the body are numerous, some of these are as follows:–

- It counteracts night blindness and helps weak eyesight—it helps in the formation of the retina in the eye.
- It helps the respiratory system to fight off infection.
- It helps in the formation of bones, healthy skin, hair, teeth and gums.
- When applied externally it helps in the healing of acne, impetigo and all skin affections, including boils and carbuncles.
- It can also help in the treatment of lung problems such as emphysema (see p. 8).
- It promotes the health of the thyroid gland, which regulates growth hormones.

Excessive consumption of vitamin A is dangerous. To produce toxic effects it is necessary to take 100,000 International Units daily for adults, and in the region of 18,500 International Units for children. Expectant mothers should not take more than 10,000 units a day.

The main source of vitamin A in food is in animal and fish livers, where the vitamin is most concentrated, but it is also to be found in milk and butter, eggs and kidneys, and it is added to margarine by law. All yellow fruits are good sources of vitamin A, and so are vegetables such as carrots, cabbage and spinach. It has been noted that persons suffering from cancer of the lung, throat, mouth, oesophagus, stomach and colon are often seriously deficient in vitamin A, and it is recommended that people suffering from this disease would be well advised to increase their intake of these vegetables.

Vitamin B Complex

In my opinion, when a particular B vitamin is called for the B Complex is the obvious answer, because although there are thirteen different vitamins contained in the B Complex they are all interdependent, and if any one single B vitamin is taken it can cause a deficiency of each of the others. In addition, if you are lacking in one B vitamin you are probably lacking in all the others as well.

People lacking in vitamin B are usually depressed, irritable and tired. Very often the appetite is very poor and sometimes too there is premature greyness and thinning hair. People who perform a lot of exercise or those who have to do heavy manual labour are particularly at risk of the depletion of vitamin B in the body. Stress is also a factor, and of course the taking of alcohol and white sugar uses up this vitamin. Being water-soluble it cannot be stored by the body and therefore a daily intake is required, but there is no danger of a toxic reaction.

Vitamin B₁—Thiamine. Up to 50 per cent of thiamine can be lost in cooking—boiling, baking, toasting, so a supplement is particularly necessary. The absence of vitamin B₁ from the diet leads to the development of beriberi—a disease in which inflammation of the nerves occurs, with muscular weakness and heart fatigue. The best sources of this vitamin are wholemeal flour, bacon, liver and egg yolk, yeast and the pulses. The daily requirement is dependent among other things on the total food intake and has been estimated to be in the region of 1.4 mg for adults, 1 mg for children up to 12 years.

Vitamin B2—Riboflavin. This vitamin plays an important part in the metabolism of proteins, fats and carbohydrates in the diet—it helps break them down so that the body can use them. The main food sources are milk and other dairy products such as butter, cheese, meat. The required daily amounts vary but it is in the region of 0.5 mg per day for infants, 1.6 mg daily for teenagers and approximately 1.2 mg per day for adults. Soreness of the lips and tongue are deficiency symptoms peculiar to this vitamin, also greasy and scaly facial skin. There is no known toxic reaction, but when taking this vitamin the urine assumes a yellowish colour. This is nothing to worry about, and quite normal.

Vitamin B3. Deficiency of this vitamin produces a condition called pellagra—dermatitis sometimes accompanied by diarrhoea—and may even cause mental disturbances. It has a function similar to that of vitamin B2 in the body. The required daily amount varies between 12 and 18 mg. It is very useful in the reduction of cholesterol in the body and in arthritis. It should always be incorporated in a B Complex tablet.

Vitamin B5—Pantothenic Acid. This vitamin is to be found in many foods, but it is particularly concentrated in eggs, meat and wholegrain cereals. The exact requirements are unknown but for healthy adults approximately 10 mg daily is adequate. Deficiency of this vitamin produces numbness and tingling, abdominal and muscle cramps, headaches and weakness, also painful, burning feet.

Vitamin B6. Here again this vitamin should be taken as part of the

B Complex range. It is to be found in fish, egg yolk, nuts and seeds, cereals and some fruit and vegetables. Deficiency symptoms include sleeplessness, nervousness, irritability and mood changes. Sometimes too there is very poor appetite and loss of weight. The recommended daily dosage is no more than 50 mg.

Vitamin B12. The body can store this vitamin for a very long time, but some stomach and small intestine conditions can affect it so that the body becomes deficient. The signs and symptoms of deficiency are those of anaemia—pale skin and mucous membranes, shortness of breath and great tiredness. Damage to the nervous system can occur if the deficiency is not treated early, and this results in difficulty with walking and pronounced tingling of the hands and feet. Elderly people lacking in this vitamin can become confused—it is usually passed off as old age but in actual fact it can be a lack of vitamin B12. People with pernicious anaemia, anyone who has had part of their stomach removed and vegetarians all need extra B12.

Liver and organ meats are the best sources but brewer's yeast, eggs, butter, cheese, milk and cream also contain it, and there is a little in fish. Supplements are usually given by injection, either by the doctor, nurse or sometimes by the patient himself. The dosage depends on the condition of the patient and it is always prescribed by the patients doctor.

Vitamin C

This is especially found in fresh fruit and fresh, green vegetables, and also to a smaller extent in milk, meat and other fresh foods. Its deficiency leads to a condition known as scurvy, which includes muscular weakness, haemorrhages under the skin, swelling and inflammation of the gums, leading to loss of teeth. It can occur in babies who are fed persistently on artificial foods. The daily requirement of vitamin C is 30 mg for adults and 60 mg for children, but people suffering from colds, chest infections, diabites or cancer benefit enormously from doses of this vitamin of up to 1,000–2,000 mg daily.

Vitamin D

This vitamin is very important to growth in children, and its deficiency leads to a condition known as rickets, with softening of bones and irregular growth, swollen joints and distorted limbs and deformities of the chest. It has long been known that cod-liver oil is the chief remedy for rickets. Only a few foods contain this vitamin naturally. Fish-liver oils are rich in it, but it may be found to a lesser extent in egg yolk and milk.

It aids the absorption of calcium and phosphorus in the body and increases their amount in the blood, and thus in the bones. An overdose can result in too much calcium being maintained in the body, which causes stones to form in the kidneys or other organs. The recommended daily dosage for nursing mothers is between 400 and 800 international units, whilst for other adults it is in the region of 400 international units.

Vitamin E

This vitamin is an anti-oxidant, which means it protects fats from being destroyed in the body by oxygen. It also protects the pituitary and adrenal glands, and the sex hormones. It strengthens the heart muscle and the artery walls, it increases circulation and has a very beneficial value in the relief of cramps and pins and needles. Combined with lecithin—which is a fat emulsifier—it has been known to assist in the relief of varicose veins.

Vitamin E is important for the skin. When it is applied externally to wounds the healing process is speeded up, and it is also known to minimize wrinkles, scar tissue and stretch marks. In the treatment of burns, if applied immediately, it is invaluable. I also give vitamin E for menopausal symptoms, such as nerves, hot flushes, sweating and depression—in these conditions it is invaluable. It is also said to assist fertility.

The vitamin has no known toxic effects, but for people suffering from rheumatic heart conditions, high blood pressure or angina or any circulatory problems it is wise to start with a fairly low intake. There is no recommended daily dosage for vitamin E but it is in the region of between 100 and 400 international units for the average person. It is a fat-soluble vitamin, which means that it can't be absorbed by the body unless fat is present, and bile is also necessary. The presence of selenium in the diet enhances the action of vitamin E and increases its effectiveness. The best sources are wheatgerm (the outer husk of the wheat), vegetable oils and whole grain cereals. It is not normally destroyed in cooking but it is reduced by the refining of food.

Minerals and Trace Elements

Minerals are elements necessary to life. We need two kinds—the macro-minerals and the trace elements. The macro-minerals are required in large dosages of several hundred milligrammes per day, and they are involved in the building of bones and cells amongst other vital functions. The trace elements are those we only require small amounts of daily, and these include iron, zinc, iodine, selenium, magnesium, chromium, molybdenum, sulphur, cobalt. All these minerals and trace elements are dependant on each other for proper functioning, and inter-actions between proteins, vitamins, minerals and trace elements are always going on.

Calcium

Calcium is one of the macro-minerals, and is required by the body in the formation of bones and teeth, and for the health of the hair, eyes, skin and nails. This mineral is very often lacking in the elderly, and indeed from middle age onwards. A lot of people in their later years suffer from brittle bones—a condition known as osteoporosis. Ridged nails and dry skin are symptoms of a lack of this mineral, and the right calcium intake for the individual is most important.

Good dietary sources of calcium are milk and milk products, green vegetables, nuts, seeds and peas, beans and lentils. I have found when treating arthritis and rheumatism, with which I get excellent results, that nearly all my patients suffer calcium deficiency, and a good natural supplement according to the individual's deficiency produces quick results. The recom-mended daily dosage varies between 500 mg and 1,500 mg.

Phosphorus

This helps calcium in the formation of bones and teeth, and is involved in the storage and release of energy—it is usually to be found along with calcium in the diet.

Potassium

This is present in every cell in the body and is a very important factor in the health and correct functioning of the heart muscles and nerves. It is found in fresh fruits, vegetables and unprocessed grain.

When a person is deficient in potassium the appetite is poor, and mental and muscle fatigue are apparent. An irregular heartbeat may be found on examination, and sometimes the patient complains of cramps in the muscles, swelling of the tissues, headaches and pains in the joints. The patient may also be very depressed. Diabetics and people on steroids can lose potassium very quickly, and other diseases may cause a deficiency. Diuretics (substances which increase the amount of urine produced) deplete the potassium in the body.

Sodium

Sodium chloride is common salt, and is an essential item in the diet. It also has medicinal uses. It is used to make normal saline solution which is injected into the blood vessels to replace fluid lost by bleeding, and for other purposes. A little salt in a glass of water makes an excellent gargle or mouth wash. A tablespoon in a glass of water serves as an emetic. A pound of common salt to a bath of hot water is often used to relieve pain in chronic joint disorders.

Working in very hot environments, which cause excessive sweating, can bring about a loss of sodium in the body. Deficiency symptoms include dizziness, cramps, nausea, vomiting and sometimes collapse. In these instances sodium chloride must be administered either as a drink or in tablet form.

Magnesium

This mineral helps in the absorption of sodium, calcium and

potassium. It is found in leafy green vegetables, nuts, soya beans and very often in tap water. Deficiency symptoms of magnesium can all be related to those of sodium, potassium and calcium. There is weakness, loss of appetite, tiredness, depression, numbness and tingling, cramps, muscle incoordination, sleeplessness and constipation. An irregular heartbeat is evident.

Supplements of magnesium and vitamin B6 have been found extremely beneficial in the treatment of kidney-stones. Any diuretic will cause a loss of magnesium in the body and this applies in no small measure to the action of alcohol, which increases the amount of urine. Diabetics are also at risk because of the high amount of urine they pass. Calcium and magnesium work very closely together, and any supplementation should be one part of magnesium to two parts calcium.

Iron

Iron deficiency is very common today and anyone who does not have a good nourishing diet is at risk. The patient usually has a very good idea if he is anaemic—he feels tired and listless, the appetite is poor and he often catches one infection after another. A visit to the doctor will confirm his fears. Mild anaemia is easy enough to correct. A good natural iron tablet—50 mg daily, 500 mg vitamin C to help absorption, is all that is needed. In a very short time a feeling of well-being returns and all is well.

Tea and coffee have been known to hinder the absorption of iron, and the stronger the tea and coffee the greater the problem. Whenever possible iron preparations should be given by mouth. The main form in which it is used is ferrous sulphate. This can cause irritation of the gastro-intestinal tract and should therefore always be taken after meals. It sometimes produces a tendency to constipation.

Zinc

Deficiency of zinc results in lack of growth, slow sexual development and anaemia. Deficiency also contributes to skin problems, diabetes and diarrhoea. Oysters are reputed to be a rich source of zinc, and so are bananas. It has many uses, the most common being zinc sulphate in the form of eye drops to treat conjunctivitis. Zinc oxide, zinc sterate and zinc carbonate are used in dusting powders and ointments. Zinc and castor oil ointment is well known in the treatment of napkin rash. It is slightly astringent and very soothing in its action and is much used in inflammation of the skin.

When there is severe zinc deficiency the immune system suffers, and we cannot fight off the various infections that we come into contact with day by day. This leads to all sorts of problems—the appetite becomes impaired, and so do senses of taste and smell, and sometimes the patient can't sleep. Gastric problems can occur and perhaps even diabetes. Wounds are slow to heal and the patient may go from one infection to the next.

Those particularly at risk from a zinc deficiency are vegetarians, people with anorexia nervosa, those on weight-reducing diets, people who suffer with coeliac disease and those on high fibre diets. People taking penicillamine for arthritis need to take zinc, and so does anybody with bowel disease or any intestinal disease. Diuretics drain zinc from the body, so it is vital for those who drink a lot of alcohol. Anybody with cancer needs zinc to promote the health of the immune system. Zinc is also essential for the correction of an impaired sense of taste, and it has also been found that night blindness can sometimes be due to a deficiency of zinc.

I have found in the running of this clinic that zinc supplementation reduces the joint swelling and morning stiffness in the vast majority of my arthritic patients. I have also found that Crohn's disease responds well to zinc supplementation in conjunction with other vitamins and minerals. As most arthritic patients are taking drugs when they come to this clinic—a lot of them are on penicillamine and steroids, which especially deplete the absorption of zinc in the body—and on examining the nails and doing the zinc test I find they are deficient. A course of zinc helps enormously to bring about a feeling of well-being.

Iodine

Iodine is extensively used in medicine in various preparations.

The strong tincture is painted on the skin as a counter-irritant. It is also used as an antiseptic paint to prepare the skin for operation. It can also be painted on chilblains or on the gum after it has been dried for the relief of toothache. Iodine ointment is used in various skin diseases requiring stimulating or antiseptic treatment.

Preparations of iodine are given for chronic bronchitis, asthma and sometimes too for chronic joint complaints. To avoid irritations of the stomach preparations of iodine should always be taken well-diluted and after food. Iodine is normally present in the body in organic combination in the secretion of the thyroid gland. It is added to all cooking salt.

Chromium

Chromium has recently been discovered to be necessary in the control of blood sugar. It is usually found in wholewheat bread, brewer's yeast and cheese.

Selenium

It seems that a deficiency of selenium may contribute to cancer and heart attacks, alopaecia, tooth decay, loss of appetite and weight loss. Sometimes the nervous system can be affected, with pins and needles, cramp, numbness and pain in the hands and feet. Vitamin E supplements should always be taken with selenium as one enhances the effects of the other in the body.

There are many more lesser-known minerals, but the above should convey to the reader how important it is to have a correct balance of vitamins and minerals each day. The only way this can be effected is by supplementing the diet each day with a good multi-vitamin and multi-mineral formation in a natural tablet. If any irregular symptoms occur and persist for a long time a naturopath or doctor should be consulted and the root cause investigated. The norm should be a healthy mind in a healthy body, and any deviation from that is abnormal and should be seen to by a competent practitioner.

Protein

Proteins are referred to as flesh-forming foods, because they are used in the body to build protoplasm, a substance which makes up the essential material of animal and plant life. In the process of digestion the complex proteins are split up into substances known as amino acids. These are absorbed from the digestive tract and carried in the blood to the body cells. The elements contained in proteins are carbon, hydrogen, oxygen and nitrogen.

A healthy person requires a relatively small amount of protein. Most cheeses contain a high protein content, and milk is also quite high in protein. Beef, veal, mutton, lamb, chicken and fish, especially smoked herring, contain high quantities. Vegetables and fruit are quite low in this commodity, so vegetarians should take instant protein powder, available from health food shops.

Conclusion

There is a growing interest among people generally in the problems of health and how good health can be achieved without taking the many and varied drugs that cause so many side effects. I feel this interest should be extended and deepened, as there is no subject about which the public could more profitably be informed.

Throughout this book the practical needs of the sufferer have been kept in mind and every effort has been made to help the patient to help himself. Many of the diseases that affect us are by no means inevitable and could be prevented by the adoption of the rules for general good health. Considerable responsibility for taking measures designed to promote health must be assumed by the individual, and the majority of people have still to learn how to keep healthy when they have attained that state. However, training and experience are needed for the correct treatment of illness and I feel that a correct diagnosis made by the patient's doctor is most important. The manifestations of disease are frequently elusive and puzzling and a correct interpretation can only be made by one whose business it is to deal with sickness.

In the treatment of minor illnesses, however, it is very desirable that reliance, when possible, should be placed on a correction of habits as regards diet, exercise, rest and so on, rather than on drugs.

Appendix 1

Recommended Daily Requirements of Vitamins and Minerals

Vitamins

Vitamin A	4,000 I.U. (International Units). Children and pregnant women require more.
Vitamin B1	0.5 mg per 1000 calories, increasing during pregnancy to 2 mg.
Vitamin B2	0.5–3 mg, more during pregnancy and lactation.
Vitamin B3	approx 12–18 mg.
Vitamin B6	minimum 2–3 mg.
Vitamin B12	varies, but always given under medical supervision.
Vitamin C	30 mg for adults, 60 mg for children.
Vitamin D	400 I.U. for adults, 400–800 for infants and nursing mothers.
Vitamin E	100–400 I.U.

Minerals

Calcium	Children 500 mg.
	Adolescents 700 mg.
	Adults 500–900 mg.
	Pregnant or nursing mothers 1,200 mg.
Iron	15–20 mg.
Zinc	100–400 mg

No recommended daily amounts have been established for trace elements.

Appendix 2

Vitamins and Food

We all need knowledge as to where to find the vitamins and minerals necessary for our requirements. Here I shall endeavour to give the best food sources of the individual vitamins and minerals.

Vitamin A

Liver, carrots, potatoes, broccoli, kale, spinach, endive, melon, peas, asparagus, green beans, egg, sweetcorn, lettuce.

Vitamin B₁—Thiamine

Sunflower seeds, brewer's yeast, soya flour, beef liver, rolled oats, brown rice, wholewheat flour, navy beans, chick peas, kidney beans, split peas, asparagus, rye flour, soya beans.

Vitamin B₂—Riboflavin

Beef liver, kidney, heart, milk, yoghurt, broccoli, soya beans, cheese.

Vitamin B₃—Niacin

Most fish, chicken, beef, brewer's yeast, peanuts, brown rice, wholewheat flour, all dried beans.

Vitamin B₆

Fish, cod, halibut, salmon, mackerel, chicken, beef, brewer's yeast, wholewheat flour, brown rice.

Vitamin B₁₂

Cheese, beef, lamb, chicken, yoghurt, eggs, liver, organ meats, butter, milk and cream.

Vitamin C

Fresh oranges, strawberries, tomatoes, grapefruit, lemons,

potatoes, broccoli, cauliflower, peppers, blackberries, cherries, cabbage, spinach, brussels sprouts.

Vitamin D

Cod-liver oil & halibut-liver oil, herring, mackerel.

Vitamin E

Wheat germ oil, wholegrain cereals, vegetable oils, cod-liver oil, corn, soya and peanut oil.

Index

Acid-free diet 15, 16, 17, 36, 68, 69, 71–2, 74
Acids 3, 15, 16, 68, 69, 71, 72, 73
Acne 39
Adenoids 3
Allergy 10, 37, 38, 78
Anaemia 23, 24, 27, 32–4, 41, 42, 54, 69, 73
Angina 65–6
Antibiotics 10, 34
Arthritis 1, 12, 15, 36, 48, 68–79
Aspirin 46, 68
Asthma 9–13
Attitude 17

Backache 47–9
Baldness 42–3
Bed sores 75–6
Biliousness 26
Body fat 27–9
Boils 40
Bright's disease 63, 79
Bronchitis 5–9, 13, 63, 65
    chronic 8–9
Burns 76

Calcium 41, 50, 87
Cancer 16–17
Carbuncles 4
Castor oil 21, 77
Catarrh 3, 4, 8
Chicken pox 66
Chromium 19, 91
Circulation 30

Cod-liver oil 8
Cold sores 3
Colds 3–5
Colic 19–21
Colitis 16
Complementary medicine 2
Constipation 19, 20, 22, 23–6, 27, 30, 31, 33, 48, 49, 54, 56
    in children 26
Cough mixture 7, 65
Coughs 6, 7
Cramp 49–52, 69
Cystitis 35–6

Dandruff 42
Dermatitis 38–9
Diabetes 4, 17–19
Diarrhoea 13, 19, 21–3, 34, 63, 77
    in children 21–2
Diet
    acid-free 15, 16, 17, 36, 68, 71–2, 74
    balanced 28–9
    fluid 7
    fruit-juice 4
    faulty 6, 15, 16, 20, 21, 22, 23, 32, 37, 45, 56, 81
    high fibre 31, 57
    wholefood 15, 16, 17, 24, 26, 33, 36, 39, 41, 46, 56, 60, 63
    for convalescents 7, 14, 16, 22, 63
    for ulcers 15

97

Dietary fibre 29
Diverticulitis 16, 70
Dizziness 57
Drug reactions 13
Drugs 1, 2, 93

Earache 77
Eczema 4, 38
Emphysema 8, 27
Enema 20, 22, 25, 32
Epilepsy 58
Epsom salts 7, 9, 46, 70
Exercise 5, 17, 19, 23, 24, 27, 30, 48, 53, 54, 56, 59

Fever, symptoms 61–2
Fibrositis 46–7
Food poisoning 77–8
Friar's balsam 7

Gargles 4
Garlic capsules 8, 9
Grapes 11, 64
Gripe water 20

Haemorrhoids 31
Headache 78
Heart disease 52–5
Heartburn 78
Hiccoughs 57
Honey 4, 10, 36, 41, 61, 70

Indigestion 48, 54, 58, 79
Insect bites 78
  stings 79
Iodine 90–91
Iron 25, 34, 41, 50, 58, 65, 89
Itching 78

Jaundice 16

Laxatives 25, 26, 33, 37, 70
Lethargy 5
Lumbago 46, 47

Magnesium 88–9

Massage 46, 47, 48, 50–52, 54, 74, 79
Measles 62–3
  German 66–7
Migraine 79
Minerals 87–91, 94
Molasses 70
Multi-minerals 35, 36, 47, 58, 69, 81
Multi-vitamins 7, 10, 31, 35, 36, 41, 52, 53, 54, 58, 69, 81
Mumps 66
Muscular rheumatism 45, 46–7

Natural medicine 13
Nervous breakdown 58–60
Nettle rash 37

Obesity 27–9
Olbas oil 4, 7, 9, 14, 49, 57, 66
Osteopath 11, 47
Overwork 6
Oxygen 5

Palpitations 57
Phosphorus 88
Piles 24, 31, 48
Pneumonia 10, 13, 63
Potassium 10, 46, 88
Protein 92

Rheumatism 46, 48, 53, 56
Rhinophyma 40

Salmonella 77
Scabies 43–4
Scalds 76
Scarlet fever 63–4
Selenium 91
Slipped disc 47
Smoking 8, 17, 39, 40, 56
Sodium 88
Sprains 51, 79
Stomach-ache 80
Strains 45–6
Stress 59–60, 83
Supplements 81–92 & throughout

Thrush 34
Toothache 80

Ulcers
    stomach 15, 16, 24, 46, 70
    varicose 30, 31

Varicose veins 24, 30–31, 55
Vick 7, 9, 14
Vinegar, cider 4, 6, 36, 37, 61,
    70, 78
Vitamins 82–7, 94–6 &
    throughout
    A 82–3 & throughout
    B complex 83–5 & throughout
    C 85 & throughout
    D 86 & throughout
    E 86–7 & throughout

Whooping cough 8, 64

Yoghurt 35

Zinc 9, 36, 39, 89–90